A SHORT DESCRIPTION OF THE GLUCOSE REVOLUTION: THE POWER OF BALANCING YOUR BLOOD SUGAR

Dr. Cyrus Khambatta Spencer

1

TABLE OF CONTENTS

1

WHAT IS GLUCOSE

The Greek word for "sweet" is where the English term "glucose" comes from. Glucose is a type of sugar that serves as fuel for the body and originates from the food we eat. It is conveyed through the bloodstream into our cells and thus known as blood glucose or blood sugar. A hormone called insulin transports glucose from the bloodstream to the cells, where it is used as fuel and stored.

Blood glucose levels are higher than usual in people with diabetes. They either don't produce enough insulin or their cells don't respond to it properly.

A glucose molecule has six carbon atoms and an aldehyde group. As such, it can be referred to as a simple sugar.

Due to the fact that it has 6 carbon atoms and one aldehyde group, it is also known as dextrose and aldohexose. It can be open either as a ring or an open chain structure. In animals, it is usually produced in the liver and kidneys. It is also present in plants. The kind of glucose that naturally exists is D-glucose. It can exist in liquid or solid form. It is also soluble in acetic acid and water. It tastes delicious and has no odor. German scientist "Andreas Marggraf" extracted glucose from raisins in 1747. Jean Baptiste Dumas first used the term glucose in 1838.

2

HOW VITAL IS GLUCOSE TO HUMAN HEALTH

One of the most crucial elements of human health is glucose. It fuels our energy and gives us the stamina to get through the day. For energy synthesis, tissue healing, and regular metabolic function, our bodies depend on glucose. The most fundamental bodily functions, including walking, thinking, and even breathing, require glucose.

Foods like fruits, vegetables, cereals, and dairy products include glucose, a simple sugar. Other carbs, including starch and glycogen, are broken down by the body into glucose and other smaller molecules. The blood then carries the glucose to the body's cells after it has been absorbed. Once in the cells, glucose is either consumed for energy or stored as glycogen for later use as a source of energy in the liver and muscles. The body needs glucose for energy, metabolism, and the healthy operation of organs like the brain, heart, and muscles.

The major consumer of glucose is the brain, which needs consistent levels all day. The ability of the body to change other forms of sugar into glucose when necessary enables this. When blood glucose levels are low, the body releases glycogen that has been stored and turns proteins and lipids into glucose as a substitute energy source.

When blood glucose levels go too low, we get tired, lightheaded, and possibly disoriented. Diabetes, a disorder in which the body is unable to maintain a normal blood sugar level, can also be indicated by low glucose levels.

A healthy weight can be maintained with the help of glucose. Glucose can be turned to energy more quickly than fat and more effectively than protein since it is simple to digest. Consuming foods high in glucose can help people feel full longer and maintain a healthy weight when accompanied with a healthy diet.

For the brain to operate properly, glucose is also necessary. Acetyl-coA, your brain's primary energy source, is created in the presence of glucose. This molecule is essential for controlling neurotransmitters, hormones, and even memory.

Overall, glucose is necessary for the body to function and to be healthy. The body constantly needs it for metabolic processes including generating energy and tissue repair. Your health could be negatively impacted if glucose levels go too low, which could cause exhaustion or confusion in the brain and body.

Fortunately, the body can change other sugars into glucose when necessary to maintain stable blood sugar levels. Eating a balanced diet that includes foods high in glucose will help control your blood sugar levels and provide your body with the energy it needs for daily activities.

3

HOW GLUCOSE IS PRODUCED

IN ANIMALS

As we begin to eat, our body instantly gets to work processing glucose. We eat starches or complex carbs as meals. The body produces enzymes including salivary amylase, maltase, and sucrase that break down carbs into absorbable glucose molecules. The pancreas, which makes hormones like insulin and is essential to how our body processes glucose, assists the enzymes as they begin the breakdown process. Also, when we eat, our body triggers the production of insulin to deal with the rise in blood sugar levels.

Nevertheless, not everyone can count on their pancreas to step up and do the necessary tasks. When the pancreas does not generate insulin as it should, diabetes can result. In this instance, processing and controlling the internal glucose levels in humans requires external assistance (such as insulin injections). Another factor that contributes to diabetes is insulin resistance, which occurs when the liver continues to produce excessive quantities of glucose despite the body's insulin being present. Due to its role in glucose storage and ability to create glucose when required, the liver is a crucial organ in the regulation of blood sugar.

Insufficient insulin production may cause the body to liberate free fatty acids from its fat reserves, which can result in the condition known as ketoacidosis. As fat is broken down by the liver, waste chemicals called ketones are produced. When there is a large amount of ketones in the body, the ketones can become toxic.

IN PLANTS

The most crucial sugar that plants make for use as an energy source and in metabolic activities is glucose. Through a process known as photosynthesis, a six-carbon sugar molecule is created from light and converted into cellular energy. Green plants and other photosynthetic organisms, including algae and some bacteria, engage in photosynthesis, which enables them to convert solar radiation into chemical energy that is then stored as glucose.

The chloroplast, an organelle that houses chlorophyll, the green pigment that makes photosynthesis possible by absorbing solar radiation, is where photosynthesis takes place in plants.

Carbon dioxide and water are absorbed in the presence of light and combined with the energy from the chlorophyll to produce glucose molecules. The following equation describes how a sugar molecule, carbon dioxide, and oxygen are created during this process using carbon dioxide, water, and light energy:

$$6CO_2 + 12H_2O + Energy \rightarrow C_6H_{12}O_6 + 6O_2 + 6H_2O$$

A kind of energy known as ATP (adenosine triphosphate) is also produced during the chemical process of photosynthesis and is used by other metabolic processes in plants. The cytoplasm of the plant cell produces ATP, which is thought to be a source of energy that plants may use. The ATP is degraded for use in a variety of metabolic activities, including those involved in molecule movement within of cells, the production of supply molecules for cell processes, and metabolic processes involved in biosynthesis.

After being created, glucose is used in respiration to give the plant energy. The glucose molecule is disassembled during respiration to create ATP and other energy-producing molecules. Although this process takes place both with and without oxygen, the amount of ATP that is produced depends largely on the oxygen supply. When oxygen is present, the mitochondria break down glucose utilizing oxygen to make 36–38 ATP molecules for every glucose molecule. In the absence of oxygen, anaerobic respiration is performed, and only 2-4 ATP molecules are produced for every glucose molecule.

Additionally, glucose serves as an organic building component for the creation of other compounds including amino acids, chlorophyll, and cellulose as well as processes like secretion within plants. In some circumstances, the glucose molecules can be changed into other molecules for storage in the plant, such as fructose or sucrose.

In conclusion, the primary sugar created by plants through photosynthesis is glucose. It is utilized during procedures like respiration, cellular molecule synthesis, and storage for later use. Glucose is used by plants as an energy source and an organic building block for the production of other molecules through the processes of photosynthesis and respiration.

HOW DOES GLUCOSE ENTER OUR BODIES?

4

The primary source of energy in the majority of our cells is glucose. It is the main source of energy for the brain, neurological system, and muscles and is very necessary for the body to function properly. Although glucose is produced by our cells from the sugars and carbohydrates we eat, the only route for glucose to enter our bloodstream is through a process known as glycolysis.

Through a chemical process called glycolysis, glucose molecules are converted into easier-to-use energy molecules like pyruvate. The enzyme known as glucose-6-phosphatase is necessary for this process, which takes place in the cytoplasm of cells. The pyruvate molecules are then transferred into the mitochondria, the area of the cell that produces energy, after this process is finished. The pyruvate molecules are further broken down in the mitochondria to create ATP, which is the actual energy source for the cell.

After entering the bloodstream, glucose is used to produce energy. A large portion of the body's cells and organs use glucose as their main energy source. For instance, glucose is the primary fuel for the brain. When blood glucose levels are high, the pancreas secretes insulin, which aids in removing and storing blood glucose. Cells can use this glucose that has been stored when they require it.

Additionally necessary for muscular contraction is glucose. Muscles require energy to contract and carry out physical labor during exercise. In addition to being stored in the form of glycogen in muscle cells, glucose can be utilized directly by the muscle to make ATP. For the generation of long-term energy, glycogen is crucial.

In conclusion, glucose enters the blood stream through the glycolysis process, which relies on the enzyme glucose-6-phosphatase. It is further broken down inside the cell into pyruvate and sent to the mitochondria, where it is changed into ATP. Cells and organs like the brain and muscle cells use glucose for energy production after that. It can also be stored as glycogen. Without glucose, our cells would be unable to produce energy, which might have potentially fatal effects.

5

WHAT CAUSES HIGH BLOOD GLUCOSE IN THE MORNING?

Highs in the morning might be puzzling. After all, you haven't consumed any carbohydrates since you just spent the previous eight to nine hours sleeping. What is happening? The dawn phenomenon and waning insulin levels are the two primary causes of morning highs. The Somogyi effect, the third, far more uncommon reason, could also be the reason.

Your A1C, a measurement of your average blood glucose (blood sugar) levels over time that shows how effectively your diabetes is managed, will be minimally affected by the occasional morning spike. But, if such highs persist, they can raise your A1C to dangerous levels.

THE DAWN PHENOMENON

Hormones like cortisol and growth hormone tell the liver to increase the synthesis of glucose in the early morning, which gives you energy to wake up. In order to maintain healthy blood glucose levels, this causes the pancreatic beta cells to produce insulin. But, if you have diabetes, you might not produce enough insulin or you might be too resistant to insulin to stop the rise in blood sugar. Your levels may be higher when you wake up as a result. Diabetes types are not differentiated by the dawn phenomena. It is experienced by almost half of those with type 1 or type 2 diabetes.

WANING INSULIN

Overnight, if your insulin level drops too low, your blood sugar levels increase. The causes of the decline in insulin differ from person to person, but they most frequently happen when your long-acting insulin dose is too low or your basal (background) insulin supply on your insulin pump is set too low. Another factor is insulin duration, or how long the medicine is active in your body. Your long-acting insulin may not persist through the night if you dose it early.

THE SOMOGYI'S EFFECT

The Somogyi effect is the body's reaction to low blood sugar (hypoglycemia) throughout the night and is named after Michael Somogyi, PhD, a chemist who was the first to explain it in the

1930s. Let's say you skip supper or overindulge in insulin after dinner. Overnight, your blood sugar levels might drop too low. You awaken with high blood glucose because your body produces additional glucose to make up for the imbalance.

6

GLUCOSE SPIKES

Diabetes patients must keep an eye on their blood sugar levels to prevent increases. A person may have increased thirst, impaired vision, and headaches if their blood sugar level is high. Diabetes is a medical condition that can lead to high blood sugar levels. There is therefore the need to control it to avoid problems.

In some situations, a change in one's lifestyle might help to control blood sugar levels. Yet some people might need to take medicine.

Either the pancreas does not generate insulin in a person with diabetes, or the cells become resistant to this hormone. As a result, the glucose stays in the blood, maintaining constant high blood sugar levels. It is known as hyperglycemia.

Blood sugar rises following meals are common among diabetics. But, if a person can't control their condition, they can continue to have high blood sugar levels. This raises the risk of cardiovascular disease and other problems associated with diabetes, such as nerve damage, eyesight loss, kidney damage, and kidney issues.

SYMPTOMS

Normally, symptoms of hyperglycemia do not appear until blood sugar levels are excessive or persistently high.

Early signs of hyperglycemia include the following:

• Thirst

• Urinating often

• Distorted eyesight

• Headache

Hyperglycemia can be brought on by both type 1 and type 2 diabetes. The symptoms may arise rapidly in those with type 1 diabetes, but they tend to develop more slowly in those with type 2 diabetes.

Ketones may begin to accumulate in the blood and urine in people with type 1 diabetes when their blood sugar levels increase uncontrolled. When insulin levels are excessively low, a particular form of acid called ketones may build up in the blood.

Ketone levels that are too high might have negative effects. Some of the effects include:

• Breath that smells fruity

• Shortness of breathing

• Dry mouth

• Weakness

• Dizziness and vomiting

• Confusion

Physicians should advise patients on what to do in the event of an exceptionally high blood sugar level and when to seek medical attention.

7

CONSEQUENCES OF UNCONTROLLED BLOOD SUGAR

Uncontrolled glucose levels have a number of long-term effects that result in a variety of disorders, as listed below.

• Heart conditions

• Neuropathy

• Infection of the skin

• Blindness

• Profound dehydration

• Issues with the joints and extremities, particularly the foot

• Coma

Diabetes-related disorders including diabetic ketoacidosis and hyperglycemic hyperosmolar syndrome also have dangerous side effects.

Individuals who are concerned that they may have diabetes are encouraged to consult a doctor right away.

8

MANAGEMENT OF BLOOD SUGAR SPIKES

Each kind of diabetes requires frequent blood glucose monitoring and management to avoid increases. The following tactics may be useful for them:

MONITORING THE LEVEL OF ONE'S BLOOD SUGAR

It's crucial to know when to seek emergency medical attention or call a doctor. Advanced health issues may result from severe blood sugar increases.

Blood sugar levels should be checked right away by anyone exhibiting hyperglycemia symptoms. Within two hours of having a meal, if the reading is greater than 180 milligrams per deciliter, they should call the doctor. Recording blood sugar readings in a notebook and scanning for trends, such rises in blood sugar every morning, may also be helpful. If this occurs, it may be time to talk to the doctor about modifying the insulin dosage. A doctor can suggest taking insulin at mealtimes if blood sugar levels are routinely high after meals.

Furthermore, be sure to take this notebook with you when you go to the doctor. The results may be reviewed by the doctor, who can then suggest making any required changes to the management strategy.

MAINTAINING A HEALTHY LIFESTYLE

A person with type 2 diabetes may be able to keep their blood sugar levels constant without the use of medication in the early stages of the disease.

Frequent, light to moderate-intensity exercise reduces blood glucose levels by using up part of the extra glucose.

The amount of glucose in the body as well as the danger of spikes can both be decreased by adhering to a low Glycemic Index (GI) diet and strict portion control. The GI rating shows how much the carbohydrates in a particular food will impact blood sugar levels.

Crackers, popcorn, and bagels are examples of foods having a high GI, which is defined as a score of 70 or greater. Barley, bulgur, maize, and sweet potatoes are examples of low GI foods, which have a score of 55 or below.

Those who have type 1 diabetes have to make an effort to live a healthy lifestyle. Unfortunately, these people will also require lifelong supplement with insulin.

Unfortunately, these people will also require lifelong supplement with insulin.

USING SMART PUMPS AND DRUGS

One should inform their prescribing doctor if strictly adhering to a medicine and food program does not stop these increases from happening. Very likely, the doctor will change the prescription.

Anybody receiving insulin or non-insulin medications must adhere to certain schedules in order to control their diabetes.

To deliver continuous, scheduled insulin dosages, a variety of pumps and smart pumps are available. These gadgets deliver low-level insulin to control blood sugar levels while you sleep and fast. Those with type 1 diabetes use them more frequently than those with type 2 diabetes.

Smart pumps may react to blood sugar rises by connecting to a continuous glucose monitor, thereby acting as an artificial pancreas. Nonetheless, human inputs are still required during meals with all pumps.

HOW TO CHECK YOUR GLUCOSE LEVELS

There are several methods you may use to monitor your blood glucose levels. They consist of:

• Fasting glucose test: Following an 8–12-hour fast, a member of the medical care team will draw a sample of blood to determine your blood sugar level. A fasting blood sugar level of 70 to 99 mg/dL is regarded as normal by the World Health Organization (WHO), whereas a reading of 100 to 125 mg/dL denotes prediabetes or impaired glucose tolerance and a reading of 126 mg/dL or higher denotes diabetes. Remember that reference ranges might differ from lab to lab. The same is true for biological sex and age.

• HbA1c: This blood test assesses how much glucose is bonded to hemoglobin, the component of red blood cells that transports oxygen throughout the body. This result essentially represents your average blood glucose levels over the last three months. Red blood cells have a lifespan of about 120 days. The outcomes are shown in percentages, with a typical range being less than 5.7%. HbA1c readings between 5.7 and 6.4% percent are indicative of prediabetes, whereas readings of 6.5% or more are indicative of diabetes.

• Continuous glucose monitoring (CGM): This technique involves inserting a small sensor beneath the skin, typically on the arm or belly, which measures your blood sugar every few minutes and sends the results to a computer, smartphone, or tablet. You may wear a GCM all the time or only for a short while, but you'll need to switch out the censor every few days.

9

THE GLUCOSE CURVE:

KNOWING YOUR BODY'S REACTION TO FOOD

For those who want to comprehend and manage their blood sugar levels, a glucose curve is crucial. This particular evaluation of how your body responds to food consumption is crucial to the effective control of diabetes. You can lower your overall risk of problems from diabetes by learning to control your carbohydrate intake and spot significant trends in your blood sugar levels.

The glucose curve shows how your body reacts to various carbohydrate types. It records on a graph the amount of blood sugar your body has after consuming various kinds of food. Additionally, it reveals the speed at which your body breaks down carbs and the time it takes for your blood sugar levels to recover to normal. You can improve your overall blood sugar control by changing your diet and lifestyle by having a better understanding of the glucose curve.

An ideal glucose curve would show a consistent rise and fall in blood glucose levels following a meal. This curve, however, may take on a different shape for some individuals. A glucose curve can show a broad peak shortly after eating, extended recovery times for post-meal glucose levels, or even differences between lunch and dinner.

HOW TO DETERMINE YOUR GLUCOSE CURVE

By routinely checking your blood glucose levels throughout the day, you can figure out your glucose curve. To do this, go to a pharmacy and buy a blood glucose meter and glucose test strips, then do the test as directed. Blood glucose levels should be checked frequently throughout the day, including before meals, 1-2 hours after eating, in the middle of the night, and before and after physical activity. You can develop a curve that displays the patterns of your glucose levels over time by keeping track of the findings. If necessary, a doctor or diabetes educator can offer assistance in interpreting the findings and suggest a course of action.

Most people can also track and monitor this information using smartphone apps like the Glucose Buddy or MyFitnessPal apps. These apps enable users to record their outcomes and track their development over time.

Your ability to monitor your health over time and take proactive measures to maintain or improve it as necessary depends on having a reliable way to assess your blood sugar levels. Additionally, monitoring a glucose curve might assist you in making better dietary and lifestyle choices to maintain appropriate glucose levels. In certain situations, people with chronic medical diagnoses like diabetes should speak with a doctor for tailored guidance.

In conclusion, knowing your glucose curve can help you better manage your diabetes. You can work with your doctor to modify your food and lifestyle after spotting patterns in your glucose curve. You can take the required actions to enhance your overall glucose levels and lower your risk of complications from diabetes with careful monitoring and effective diabetic management.

10

HOW TO FLATTEN YOUR GLUCOSE CURVE

EATING THE CORRECT DIET

Your glucose curve can "flatten" with a diet that carefully manages the timing and sequence of the items you consume. To avoid glucose spikes and drops and to maintain your body functioning like an efficient machine, this idea can be applied to meals and snacks.

Every food you eat contains carbohydrates that will impact your blood sugar levels, but some are broken down and absorbed more quickly than others. When carbohydrates from fast digested foods with a high glycemic index are ingested on an empty stomach, they might cause your blood sugar to rise quickly. On the other side, slow-digesting and slow-absorbing foods, like those high in fiber, can lessen the risk of glucose spikes and low blood sugar.

It's crucial to balance the high- and low-glycemic food groups in each meal and snack in order to maintain stable blood sugar levels and a healthy body. A starchy food, such as oats, potatoes, pasta, or whole-grain bread, should be added after a protein, such as lean meat, fish, or nuts, which are absorbed more slowly. Your glucose levels can be stabilized by consuming carbohydrates and slowly digested proteins together. To your meals and snacks, try to add some unsweetened fruits and veggies. These usually contain fewer carbohydrates and offer fiber, vitamins, and other necessary nutrients. Slowing the absorption of carbohydrates can also be accomplished by consuming a small quantity of healthy fats such those found in avocados, olive oil, nuts, and seeds.

It's also crucial to keep in mind that your daily dietary decisions will have an impact on how much glucose you have throughout the day. To avoid a mid-morning collapse in energy or glucose levels, eat a wholesome breakfast that includes protein and healthy fats, for instance. Your body can avoid going too low on energy and glucose by eating a variety of small, balanced meals and snacks throughout the day.

Your glucose levels can be kept in check by eating the proper foods at the proper times throughout the day. To ensure that your body receives the nutrients it requires, eat a balanced diet that includes proteins, complex carbohydrates, fruits, vegetables, and healthy fats. This will not only help you keep your blood sugar levels stable, but it will also help you have the energy and endurance you need to get through your daily tasks.

ADDING GREEN

Foods high in dietary fiber include green starters. These can be steamed veggies, fresh salads, or other green foods. These green starts' soluble fiber can help maintain more stable blood sugar levels throughout the day by slowing the pace at which glucose is released into the system.

Therefore, having a green starter before every meal can aid in lowering your glycemic reaction following food. This can stop the sharp spikes and drops in blood sugar that can be particularly harmful to your health. Green beginnings can also make you feel satisfied for a longer period of time, which can help you better control your appetite and lessen cravings throughout the day.

When it comes to including a green starting in all of your meals, there are a variety of delectable and healthful possibilities. The majority of green vegetables can be utilized to create a delicious and nutrient-dense sauce or soup because they are so nutrient-dense and low in calories. Excellent options include kale, cabbage, broccoli, spinach, lettuce, and celery. Additionally, you can use your imagination to create salads with spirulina, dulse seaweed, or even edible flowers. Find your favorite greens by experimenting with different mingling and matching combinations.

You should think about drinking green beginnings in addition to adding them to every meal. Wheatgrass juice, cucumber and celery juices, as well as green smoothies, are all delicious low-calorie substitutes for snacks and desserts.

You can help to balance your blood sugar levels, improve your health, and have fewer cravings and hunger sensations by including a green beginning in every of your meals. So make it a habit and check to see that your regular diet contains enough.

PUT AN END TO COUNTING CALORIES

Instead of just counting calories, our goal in this book is to flatten your glucose curve. We must first examine how glucose affects our health in order to comprehend why this is so crucial. The body uses glucose as its main energy source and it plays a role in many bodily functions. Additionally, it is necessary for healthy cellular activity and is crucial for people with diabetes.

Our bodies convert the food we eat into glucose. The cells in our body then receive this glucose and utilise it to fuel themselves. Unfortunately, high blood sugar levels brought on by an excess of glucose in the blood can induce long-term cell damage. Diabetes problems may emerge if untreated.

It's more crucial to concentrate on flattening your glucose curve in order to avoid significant blood glucose spikes. This entails controlling the rate of glucose release in your body to prevent sharp spikes and troughs. You can avoid developing diabetes by doing this, which helps to reduce cell damage.

Quitting counting calories is the most effective approach to flatten your glucose curve. Focus on eating real, whole foods instead. High-fiber, high-protein, and high-healthy fat meals will maintain your blood sugar levels constant and your body functioning at its best. Reduce your intake of processed and sugary meals as well. These can result in significant rises in your blood sugar levels and further difficulties.

You can take charge of your health and flatten your glucose curve by giving up the calories and putting more of an emphasis on eating the correct kinds of food. Long-term, this will assist you in maintaining your health and avoiding diabetic issues.

FLATTEN YOUR BREAKFAST CURVE

Breakfast has been described by many nutritionist as the most important meal of the day. It helps to stabilize your blood sugar levels and sets the tone for the rest of the day. However, for other people, a typical breakfast of toast or cereal might quickly cause blood sugar levels to increase, leaving them feeling drained and unable to concentrate.

Breakfast is crucial since it revs up your metabolism and gives you energy for the day. However, the best way to prevent increases in your blood sugar levels is to eat a balanced diet that includes the correct foods.

Combining complex carbs, lean proteins, and healthy fats makes up a balanced meal. Your blood sugar will stay constant with this combo throughout the day. Complex carbohydrates contain more dietary fiber and take longer for the body to break down, which helps keep your blood sugar levels stable. Your body receives energy from lean proteins and healthy fats, which also help you feel satisfied and avoid blood sugar spikes.

Breakfast should consist of fiber-rich carbohydrates such as oats, quinoa, sweet potatoes, and legumes as these are digested more slowly than processed carbohydrates like white bread and sugary cereals. This makes it easier to keep your blood sugar stable for extended stretches of time without a sharp increase.

Furthermore, it's crucial to include meals with a low glycemic index (GI) in your breakfast. Low GI foods are ones that digest slowly and release glucose into the system more gradually. This will assist in maintaining steady blood sugar levels. Foods with a low GI include muesli, rye bread, and porridge oats.

For your breakfast curve to stay flat and prevent sharp rises in your blood sugar levels, you must eat a combination of lean proteins and healthy fats.

Eggs, Greek yogurt, and lean ground beef are examples of lean proteins that are vital because they give your body slow-burning energy. Your body receives energy from healthy fats like avocado, almonds, and seeds while also feeling fuller for longer. These proteins and good fats can be included in smoothies, protein shakes, omelettes, scrambled eggs, and other morning dishes.

You can use a few helpful strategies to flatten your breakfast curve and maintain steady blood sugar levels throughout day.

First, to maintain stable blood sugar levels, include protein, whole grains, and healthy fat in every meal. Second, have a protein-rich breakfast to help you feel fuller longer and stave off the urge to snack in the middle of the morning.

In addition, choose smaller, more frequent meals throughout the day while being aware of portion amounts. This will assist maintain stable blood sugar levels and provide your body with the proper fuel for peak performance.

The secret to sustaining stable blood sugar levels throughout the day may lie in flattening out your breakfast curve. You may start the day with the energy you need by eating a balanced breakfast that includes the correct foods, which will prevent unexpected rises in your blood sugar. Making sure that each meal provides a balance of complex carbohydrates, lean proteins, and healthy fats is crucial. You'll be well on your way to flat-lining your breakfast curve by keeping in mind these suggestions.

INSTEAD OF A SWEET SNACK, CHOOSE DESSERT

It's not necessary for sweets and other sugary snacks to have a poor reputation when it comes to diabetes and weight management. In fact, eating dessert can assist you in controlling your blood sugar.

It's crucial to pay attention to the sort of sugar you consume and when if you're managing diabetes or obesity. In general, desserts are preferable than sugary snacks, obviously in moderation. In comparison to other sweet snacks, desserts have a more complex sugar composition, which can aid to flatten the glucose curve.

Although this is a proper aspect of digestion, the speed and form of the curve are crucial for overall health, particularly in the control of diabetes and weight. The goal is to try to keep the curve flat, or at the very least under control.

Here are some reasons why desserts are preferable over sweet snacks:

• Complex carbs, or carbohydrates with a slower rate of digestion, are frequently found in desserts. This implies that the increase and fall of glucose levels, or the glucose curve, is more gradual.

• Simple carbs or carbohydrates with a faster rate of digestion are frequently used to make sweet snacks. This results in a more abrupt glucose curve and an initial quick spike in glucose levels, which can be challenging to control for those with diabetes and obesity.

•Desserts can keep you fuller for longer stretches without requiring you to consume several snacks because they take longer to digest.

It's better to minimize sweets of any kind in light of all of this. However, choose a dessert rather than a sweet snack if you're searching for something sweet as a reward. Desserts' complex sugars can help flatten the glucose curve and improve the management of diabetes and obesity.

BEFORE EATING, GET SOME VINEGAR

In recent years, drinking vinegar before meals has gained popularity as a strategy to help control blood sugar levels in the body. The capacity of vinegar to lower the glycemic index of food can help flatten the glucose curve and maintain energy levels at a more constant rate. Vinegar also has other health advantages. In this book, we'll go over how to incorporate vinegar into your diet and how it can help flatten your glucose curve.

Health Benefits of Vinegar

Acetic acid, a substance found in vinegar, is what gives it its primary health advantage. According to research, acetic acid can be used as a sugar substitute because it prevents the bloodstream from absorbing glucose.

As a result, vinegar consumption has been associated with a number of health advantages, such as lowering blood glucose levels, reducing hunger, and boosting insulin sensitivity, all of which can aid in managing weight and blood glucose levels.

Using vinegar to flatten your glucose curve: How to get there

It's simple to get vinegar before eating, and there are many different ways to achieve it. Vinegar is most frequently used as a pre-meal condiment when combined with water or another liquid. In addition, vinegar can be eaten with food or included in marinades, sauces, and salad dressings.

It's vital to keep in mind that vinegar shouldn't be consumed excessively or on an empty stomach. It is suggested to start modest and progressively increase the dosage until you discover the one that suits you the most. However, it is advised that you speak with your doctor if you have diabetes before ingesting vinegar because it could interact poorly with any drugs you are taking.

What to Take Into Account When Getting Vinegar

It's crucial to think about the type and quality of vinegar you're ingesting when deciding how much to drink. Although white vinegar is a common option, you might also want to take into account the flavor and health advantages of other vinegars, such as apple cider vinegar, red wine vinegar, and balsamic vinegar. When using vinegar to flatten your glucose curve, it's also crucial to take the vinegar's dosage into account because a larger concentration could cause your glucose levels to drop too quickly. So a decent rule of thumb is to find the lowest vinegar content that still produces the desired result.

A great technique to flatten your glucose curve and maintain more constant energy levels is to consume vinegar before meals. When using vinegar, it's crucial to think about the type and quality you're drinking as well as the lowest vinegar concentration that still produces the intended results. You may simply add vinegar into your diet and benefit from its natural health advantages by taking into account these suggestions.

EXERCISE AFTER EATING

Your glucose curve's peaks and troughs can be more evenly distributed and better controlled with exercise. The glucose curve can be flattened by exercising right after a meal, and the other physical activities you engage in during the day help to maintain steady blood sugar levels and minimize spikes.

Anaerobic and aerobic energy systems make up the body's two primary energy systems. Lifting weights, running a sprint, and jumping are all examples of anaerobic exercise. Anaerobic exercise is important for developing strength, but research indicates that aerobic exercise is especially advantageous for regulating blood sugar levels. Understanding how to employ both types of exercise to flatten your glucose curve is crucial since different types of exercise have distinct effects on the body.

Exercise that uses oxygen to produce energy, such as walking, jogging, or biking, is a continual form of play. Because aerobic activity causes the body's fat cells to become active, it can give the body an alternate energy source, assisting in the control of blood glucose levels.

Anaerobic exercise can be beneficial if your blood glucose levels start to rise after eating. The body can release glucose by creating an energy deficit thanks to the rapid energy spikes. Anaerobic exercise can also improve insulin sensitivity, which means your body will react to insulin's actions more effectively in addition to this immediate benefit. Anaerobic exercise can therefore flatten your glucose curve and enhance your overall glucose regulation.

Recent research has also shown that aerobic exercise can flatten your glucose curve even more effectively. It lessens the likelihood of a post-meal glucose surge by delaying the release of glucose into the blood. According to studies, 30 minutes of continuous aerobic exercise after meals can help manage glucose levels more effectively than periods of inactivity.

Aim for regular aerobic activity for at least 30 minutes per day in addition to shorter bursts of anaerobic exercise to achieve the best glucose management. It's crucial to remember that exercise shouldn't take the place of other healthy habits for regulating blood sugar levels, such as eating a balanced diet and getting adequate rest. But you can incorporate exercise into your overall glucose management strategies.

In conclusion, both anaerobic and aerobic exercise can help flatten your glucose curve after eating by releasing energy from fat cells and giving your body access to a different energy source. Regular physical activity can help prevent glucose spikes and improve overall glucose management when combined with a healthy diet and lifestyle.

BONUS

30 DAYS RECIPE FOR REVERSING DIABETES

DAY 1

BREAKFAST

Oatmeal Bowl with Fresh Fruit

Ingredients:

- Diced fresh fruits like strawberries, raspberries, blueberries, peaches, and apples;

- 2 cups of rolled oats;

- 2.5 glasses of water;

- 1/2 teaspoon of salt;

- Granola

- Honey

- Coconut flakes as a garnish

Directions:

1. Start by boing the water and salt in a medium saucepan.

2. After the water has boiled, add the oats and lower the heat to a low simmer.

3. Simmer for approximately 10 minutes, occasionally stirring to prevent the oats from sticking to the bottom.

4. Transfer the softened, thoroughly cooked oats to a serving bowl.

5. Sprinkle fresh diced fruits of your choice on top of the oatmeal.

6. Top with granola, honey, and coconut flakes as desired

7. Enjoy!

SNACK

Almonds and grapes

Ingredients:

-1 cup of red grapes

-1 cup of whole almonds

-1 tablespoon of olive oil and two teaspoons of honey

Directions:

1. Set the oven to 350 degrees Fahrenheit.

2. Spread the almonds out on a baking sheet and roast them in the oven for 8 to 10 minutes.

3. Combine the honey and olive oil in a small bowl.

4. After removing the almonds from the oven, add them to the bowl and toss with the honey and olive oil mixture to coat.

5. Include the grapes in the dish and mix everything until the almonds and grapes are thoroughly coated.

6. Re-distribute the almond-grape mixture onto the baking sheet, and bake for an additional 8 minutes, or until the almonds are toasted and the grapes are just barely cooked.

7. Take the almond-grape combination out of the oven, and either reheat or cool it before serving. Enjoy!

LUNCH

Quinoa salad with roasted vegetables

Ingredients

- 1 large head of floret-cut cauliflower

- 2 large red bell peppers that have been sliced into 1-inch squares.

- 2 big carrots, sliced into half-inch pieces.

- One large red onion, sliced into wedges.

- Olive oil, 2 tablespoons

- Salt and pepper as required

- 2 cups cooked quinoa

-2 teaspoons of balsamic vinegar

-2 tablespoons of freshly chopped parsley

- 2 tablespoons of freshly chopped basil

Directions:

1. Ensure the oven is set to 400 ºF.

2. Arrange the onions, carrots, bell peppers, and cauliflower on a big baking sheet. Add salt and pepper, then drizzle with the olive oil. Coat by tossing.

3. Roast the vegetables for 20 minutes, tossing them once or twice, in the preheated oven, or until they are soft and lightly browned.

4. Combine the cooked quinoa, parsley, basil, balsamic vinegar, and veggies in a sizable bowl. Combine by tossing.

5. Present warm or cold. Enjoy!

SNACK

Celery Sticks with Hummus

Ingredients

-A bunch of celery sticks

-1 cup of ready-made hummus

-Optional: Parsley, lemon juice, or any desired toppings

Directions:

1. Wash the celery sticks and dry them. To make 2-3 inch pieces, cut them.

2. Add any optional ingredients, such as fresh parsley or a squeeze of lemon juice, to the hummus in a medium bowl.

3.Spoon 1-2 teaspoons of hummus onto each celery stick to assemble the celery sticks. Enjoy!

DINNER:

Sweet potato fries and a salmon burger

Ingredients:

- 4 skinless, boneless fillets of salmon

- 1 chopped onion

- 1/4 cup almond flour;

- 1 teaspoon garlic powder

- A half teaspoon of paprika

- 2 tablespoons of olive oil

- 1/4 teaspoon of salt

- 4 sweet potatoes

Directions:

1. Ensure the oven's temperature is set to 375 ºF.

2. Combine onion, almond flour, garlic powder, paprika, and salt in a medium bowl.

3. Shape the fish into 4 patties and sprinkle with spice.

4. In a skillet set over medium heat, warm 2 tablespoons of olive oil.

5. Brown and fully cook the salmon patties by cooking them for 5 minutes on each side.

6. Cut sweet potatoes into fries after peeling.

7. Combine sweet potatoes, oil, garlic powder, paprika, and salt in a large bowl.

8. Arrange the sweet potato fries on a baking sheet covered with parchment paper.

9. Bake for 20 minutes, turning the pan once every 10 minutes.

10. Serve sweet potato fries and salmon patties with your preferred sauces and garnishes. Enjoy!

DAY 2:

BREAKFAST

Egg and spinach scramble

Ingredients:

- 3 eggs

- 2 tablespoons of shredded cheese (optional)

- 1/4 teaspoon of salt

- 1/8 teaspoon of garlic powder

- 1 tablespoon of olive oil

- 1/4 cup of chopped spinach

- 1/4 cup of chopped onion

- 1/8 teaspoon

Directions:

1. In a medium mixing bowl, crack the 3 eggs and whisk or beat them well with a fork.

2. In a medium-sized skillet set over medium heat, warm the olive oil. When the oil is hot, add the onions and spinach, and sauté, turning regularly, for about 3 minutes, until the onions and spinach are cooked and aromatic.

3. Add the beaten eggs to the skillet and stir occasionally while you scramble the eggs with the vegetables.

4. Add the cheese (if using), salt, garlic powder, and black pepper when the eggs are almost done. Scramble the eggs consistently until they are fully done.

5. Serve hot. Enjoy!

SNACK

Whole Wheat Toast with Almond or Peanut Butter

Ingredients:

- 2 pieces of whole-wheat bread

- 2 teaspoons of almond or peanut butter

- 1 teaspoon each of honey and cinnamon

- 1 tablespoon olive oil

- 1 teaspoon nutmeg

Directions:

1. Set your toaster oven's temperature to 375 degrees.

2. Lightly toast the whole wheat bread slices until they are golden.

3. Cover the toast slices with almond or peanut butter.

4. Combine honey, cinnamon, and nutmeg in a small basin. Over the toast, drizzle the mixture.

5. Olive oil should be drizzled on the toast.

6. Lay the bread out on a baking sheet and toast it in the preheated toaster oven for 7 minutes, or until it turns golden brown.

7. Dish and savor!

LUNCH

Kale and carrot salad with avocado

Ingredients:

- 2 cups of freshly torn kale leaves

- 2 medium carrots, sliced thin

- 1/4 cup red onion, chopped

- 1 diced avocado

- 2 teaspoons of lemon juice that has just been squeezed

- Extra-virgin olive oil, 2 tablespoons

- 1/4 teaspoon of sea salt

- 1/4 teaspoon of black pepper

Directions:

1. Put the kale that has been torn up in a big basin.

2. Include the avocado, red onion, and carrots.

3. Combine the lemon juice, olive oil, sea salt, and pepper in another bowl.

4. Drizzle the salad with the dressing and toss to mix.

5. Distribute the salad among the four plates and savor.

Cinnamon-infused apple slices

Ingredients:

- 2 apples

- 2 teaspoons ground cinnamon

- 2 tablespoons of honey

-2 tablespoons Olive oil

Directions:

1. Set the oven to 350 degrees.

2. Slice each apple into 8 uniform slices, then arrange them on a baking sheet that has been oiled.

3. In a small dish, combine the olive oil, honey, and cinnamon and stir to blend.

4. Apply the mixture equally to both sides of the apple slices using a brush to spread it out.

5. Cook the apple slices in the oven for 20 minutes, or until they just begin to faintly brown.

6. Before serving, let the apple slices cool just a little. Enjoy!

DINNER
Roasted Cauliflower and Broccoli with Baked Chicken

Ingredients

- 2 big skinless, boneless chicken breasts

- Olive oil, 2 tablespoons

- 1/2 teaspoon of garlic powder

- 1/2 teaspoon oregano, dry

- Salt, 1/4 teaspoon

- 1/4 teaspoon of black pepper

- 2 minced garlic cloves

- 1 cauliflower head, divided into florets

- 1 head of broccoli with florets

- 2 tablespoons lemon juice, fresh

-2 tablespoons. avocado oil

- 1/4 tablespoons garlic powder

- 1/4 teaspoon oregano, dry

- A pinch of salt and black pepper

Directions:

1. Set the oven to 425 Fahrenheit.

2. Position chicken breasts on a baking pan covered with parchment paper. Olive oil, oregano, garlic powder, salt, and pepper should be brushed on. For fifteen minutes, roast in the oven.

3. Combine the florets of broccoli and cauliflower in a big bowl. Add avocado oil and lemon juice, then season with salt, black pepper, oregano, garlic powder, and a pinch of each.

4. Arrange the broccoli and cauliflower all around the chicken breasts on the baking sheet and put the pan back in the oven. Bake the vegetables for 15-

20 minutes, or until they are cooked through and slightly browned.

5. Serve chicken and vegetables. Enjoy!

Greek Yogurt with Berries and Nuts

Ingredients

- 32 ounces of plain Greek yogurt (fat-free)

- 1/2 cup chopped walnuts

- 1/2 cup chopped almonds

- 1 cup sliced strawberries

- 1/2 a cup of blueberries

- 2 tablespoons ground flaxseeds and 2 tablespoons honey

Directions:

1. Combine the Greek yogurt, walnuts, and almonds in a large bowl.

2. Stir the yogurt mixture after adding the strawberries and blueberries.

3. Pour the honey over the yogurt mixture and swirl to incorporate it.

4. Add the ground flaxseeds and give it one last swirl.

5. Serve and savor.

SNACK

Hummus and Carrot and Celery Sticks

Ingredients:

- 2 peeled and sliced sticks of carrots

- 2 sticks of celery, sliced into stalks

- 1/2 cup of hummus, either homemade or purchased.

Directions:

1. Peel the carrots and cut them into sticks using a vegetable peeler.

2. After washing, trim the celery stalks into sticks.

3. Arrange the celery sticks and carrots on a platter.

4. Combine the hummus in a different bowl.

5. Put a dollop of hummus on the platter with the carrot and celery sticks.

6. Dish out and savor!

LUNCH

Lentil Soup with a Side Salad

Lemon Soup

Ingredients:

- Olive oil, 2 tablespoons

- 1 big diced onion

- 2 large minced garlic cloves

- 2 sliced carrots

- 2 chopped celery stalks

- 2 cups of dry lentils

- 8 cups of vegetable stock

- Tomato paste, 2 teaspoons

- salt, 1 teaspoon

- 1/2 teaspoon pepper, black

- 1/2 teaspoon of dried thyme

- Cayenne pepper, 1/4 teaspoon

Directions:

1. In a big pot over medium heat, warm the olive oil. Add the onions and garlic, and cook for about 5 minutes, or until tender.

2. Continue to sauté for 3 more minutes after adding the carrots and celery.

3. Include the tomato paste, lentils, vegetable broth, salt, pepper, thyme, and cayenne pepper. Bring to a boil on a high heat setting.

4. Lower the heat and cook the lentils for about 20 minutes, uncovered.

5. Serve with salad.

Side Salad

Ingredients:

- 2 cups spinach or arugula

- 1 cup of cucumber slices

- 1/2 a cup of cherry tomatoes

- Olive oil, 2 tablespoons

- 1 teaspoon of apple cider vinegar

- One tablespoon of Dijon mustard

- One-fourth teaspoon sea salt

Directions:

1. Place all the ingredients in a medium bowl and stir to incorporate.

2. Serve with the lentil soup. Enjoy!

Peanut butter with banana

Ingredients:

- 1 Banana

- Peanut butter, two tablespoons

-Optional splash of almond milk

Directions:

1. Peel your banana, then cut it into 1/2-inch rounds.

2. Each slice of banana should have 1 tablespoon of peanut butter on it.

3. Arrange the slices on a dish and top with almond milk, if desired.

4. Microwave the banana slices for 30 seconds, or until they are warm.

5. Serve and savor!

Stuffed Peppers with Turkey and Brown Rice

Ingredients:

- 6 medium-sized bell peppers

- 1 lb. of lean ground turkey

- 1 sliced tiny onion

- 1 teaspoon powdered garlic

- 1/2 teaspoon cumin

- 1 tablespoon of smoked paprika

- 1/2 teaspoon of oregano

- 1/2 teaspoon salt

- 1/2 teaspoon black pepper

- 2 cups of brown rice boiled

- 1 (14.5 oz) can of chopped tomatoes with no added salt

- Tomato paste, two teaspoons

- Worcestershire sauce, two tablespoons

- Balsamic vinegar, two tablespoons

- 1/4 cup chopped fresh parsley

Directions:

1. Set the oven to 375 degrees.

2. Remove and discard the seeds and membranes from each bell pepper after cutting it in half lengthwise.

3. Put bell peppers in a 9x13-inch baking dish with the cut side facing up.

4. In a large skillet, sauté the ground turkey and onion over medium heat for 8 to 10 minutes, or until the turkey is thoroughly cooked and crumbles.

5. Add salt, pepper, oregano, cumin, garlic powder, and smoked paprika to the ground turkey.

6. Turn off the heat and add cooked brown rice, tomato paste, Worcestershire sauce, and balsamic vinegar to the mixture.

7. Lightly press the turkey and rice mixture into each half of the bell pepper.

8. Bake for 35 minutes in a preheated oven, or until bell peppers are soft.

9. Finish by garnishing with freshly cut parsley. Enjoy!

BREAKFAST

Avocado and tomato omelet with egg whites -

Ingredients:

- 2 eggs whites

- 2 tablespoons 1% milk,

- Olive oil, 1 tablespoon

- 1/2 diced avocado

- 1/4 cup chopped tomatoes

- Salt & pepper, as desired

Directions:

1. In a small dish, combine the egg whites and milk and whisk until thoroughly combined.

2. In a 10-inch nonstick skillet over medium heat, warm the olive oil.

3. Add the egg mixture to the skillet and cook for 2 minutes, or until the edges start to firm.

4. Gently fold the omelet's borders inside toward the center to form fluffy pieces.

5. Top half of the omelet with the diced avocado and tomatoes.

6. Gently fold the remaining omelet half over the tomato and avocado mixture.

7. Cook the omelet for a further 2-3 minutes on each side, or until it is thoroughly cooked.

8. Transfer to a plate and add salt and pepper as desired. Enjoy!

Fresh Fruit and Greek Yogurt

Ingredients

-2 cups of unflavored Greek yogurt

- Fresh berries, such as 8 ounces of strawberries, blueberries, blackberries, or cherries

- Honey, 2 tablespoons

- Cinnamon, 1 teaspoon

- 1/4 cup of shredded almond

Directions:

1. Greek yogurt should be put into a bowl.

2. Add a combination of the fresh berries you prefer.

3. Add cinnamon and honey.

4. Combine all the ingredients.

5. Add shredded almonds on top.

6. Keep cold for 30 minutes.

7. Enjoy!

LUNCH

Vegetables Roasted with Quinoa

Ingredients:

- 2. Cups of quinoa

- 2 -3 teaspoons olive oil

- 2 minced garlic cloves

- 1 chopped red bell pepper

- 2 sliced celery stalks

- 1 diced zucchini

- 1 diced yellow squash

- 1 teaspoon of seasoning mix

- Optional: 1/4 teaspoon red pepper flakes

- 2 cups of vegetable broth

- Salt and pepper as desired

Directions:

1. Set oven temperature to 375 degrees Fahrenheit.

2. Toss the quinoa with the Italian seasoning, crushed red pepper, olive oil, garlic, bell pepper, celery, zucchini, and squash in a sizable bowl.

3. Place the vegetables and quinoa on a baking sheet, sprinkle salt and roast for 25 minutes.

4. Bring the vegetable broth to a boil in the meantime over medium-high heat.

5. When the mixture is boiling, add the roasted quinoa and vegetables, turn the heat to low, and let it simmer for 10 minutes.

6. Serve quinoa and vegetables while it is warm. Enjoy!

SNACK

Apple Slices with Almond Butter

Ingredients:

- 2 apples

- 2 teaspoons of almond butter

- 1 pinch of Himalayan salt

- A little handful of almonds, if desired

Directions:

1. Carefully cut the apples into small slices and place aside.

2. Blend almond butter with a dash of Himalayan salt in a small bowl.

3. Cover the apple slices with almond butter and arrange them on a platter or board.

4. Garnish with almond if so desired. Enjoy!

DINNER
Tilapia in the Oven with Asparagus

Ingredients

- 4-6 fillets of tilapia

- 2 teaspoons of garlic powder

- Dried oregano, 1 teaspoon

- 1 teaspoon of dried basil

- 1 teaspoon of paprika

- 2 cups of prepared asparagus

- 2 tablespoons of olive oil

- Pepper and salt as desired

Directions:

1. Ensure the oven's temperature is set to 375 ºF.

2. Arrange the tilapia fillets on a baking pan in a single layer.

3. Combine paprika, oregano, basil, and garlic powder in a small bowl.

4. Top the tilapia with the mixture.

5. Position the asparagus around the tilapia.

6. Add some olive oil.

7. Add some salt and pepper.

8. Bake for 15 to 20 minutes in a preheated oven, or until the tilapia is fully cooked and the asparagus is soft.

9. Serve hot. Enjoy!

BREAKFAST

Oatmeal with Berries and Maple Syrup

Ingredients:

- 1 cup of rolled oats

- 1 cup of almond milk

- 3 teaspoons of maple syrup

-1/2 teaspoon of cinnamon, ground

-1/4 cup blueberries, strawberries, or raspberries, fresh or frozen

Directions:

1. Combine rolled oats, almond milk, maple syrup, and ground cinnamon in a medium saucepan.

2. Heat should be reduced to low after bringing mixture to a low to medium boil (stirring occasionally).

3. To properly cook the oats, simmer them for 10 minutes while tossing occasionally to avoid sticking.

4. After the oats are cooked, turn off the heat and let the pan cool for a couple of minutes.

5. Add the berries and mix just enough to spread them.

6. Serve warm and savor!

Dried Fruit and Nuts
Ingredients:

- 1 cup of uncooked almonds

- Walnuts, 1 cup

- 1 cup of cranberries, dried

- A one cup of dried cherries

- 1/2 cup of raisins

- Pitted dates, 1/2 cup

- Chia seeds, 1/4 cup

- a quarter cup of flaxseed

- 1/4 cup of coconut flakes, shredded (optional)

Directions:

1. Set your oven to 350 fahrenheit.

2. Place almonds, walnuts, cranberries, cherries, raisins, dates, chia seeds, and flaxseed on baking sheet.

3. Roast in a preheated oven for 10 to 15 minutes, or until the fruit begins to shrivel and the nuts begin to smell toasted.

4. Remove from the oven, then allow to cool.

5. After the mixture has cooled, add the coconut shreds (if preferred) and combine all the ingredients in a bowl.

6. Keep in the fridge for up to a month in an airtight container.

7. Enjoy your tasty and nutritious blend of nuts and dried fruit!

Regular eating of nuts and dried fruit helps lower blood pressure.

LUNCH

Spinach-and-Chickpea Salad Wrap
Ingredients:

- Olive oil, 2 tablespoons

- 2 minced garlic cloves

- 2 cups rinsed and drained cooked chickpeas

- 1/4 teaspoon cumin

- 1/4 teaspoon coriander

- 1/4 teaspoon of chili powder

- Salt and freshly ground black pepper as desired.

- 1/4 cup of finely minced fresh parsley

- 2 finely sliced green onions

- Juice made from 1/2 lemon

- 2 cups of fresh spinach leaves

- 4 tortillas made of whole wheat

Directions:

1. In a medium skillet over medium-high heat, warm the olive oil.

2. After adding the garlic, add 1 minute of frequent stirring.

3. Include the cooked chickpeas along with the cumin, coriander, and chili powder. Add salt and pepper to taste. Stirring occasionally, cook the chickpeas for 3 to 4 minutes, or until they are heated through.

4. Remove from heat and toss in lemon juice, parsley, and green onions.

5. To put the wraps together, place some spinach leaves in the middle of each tortilla. Add equal

portions of the chickpea mixture on top, roll up the tortilla securely by folding the sides in.

6. Either serve warm or keep in the fridge for up to two days.

Hummus with Carrot and Celery Sticks

Ingredients :

- Cut two cups of celery stalks into 3-inch chunks.

- Cut two cups of carrots into 3-inch chunks.

- 1 cup of hummus

Directions:

1. Set the oven to 350 degrees.

2. Arrange the carrot and celery sticks on a baking pan covered with parchment paper.

3. Bake the vegetables for 20 to 25 minutes, or until they are soft and just beginning to color.

4. Put some hummus on the side and serve the vegetables. Enjoy!

Turkey Burgers and Fries made Of Sweet Potatoes

Ingredients:

-1 pound ground turkey meat

-1 egg

- 2 teaspoons of almond meal.

- 1/4 teaspoon sea salt

- 1 teaspoons of garlic powder

- Black pepper, 1/2 teaspoon

- Olive oil, two tablespoons

- 2 slices of sliced sweet potatoes

Directions:

1. Prepare a baking sheet with parchment paper and preheat the oven to 425 degrees F.

2. Mix the ground turkey, egg, almond meal, sea salt, garlic powder, and black pepper in a medium bowl until well-combined.

3. Divide the mixture into four patties and arrange them on the baking pan.

4. Drizzle olive oil over the sweet potato fries and toss to coat. On the baking sheet where the burgers are placed, spread the fries.

5. Bake the burgers for 25 to 30 minutes, turning them over halfway through. The fries have to be crispy and golden brown.

6. Put the sweet potato fries with the burgers and eat up!

DAY 6:

BREAKFAST

Bowl of Smoothie with Acai Berries

Ingredients:

- 1 cup of berries, akai

- 1 banana

- 1 cup of blueberries, frozen

- Almond milk, half a cup

- Honey, 2 tablespoons

- Cinnamon, half a teaspoon

- Chia seeds, 1/4 cup

- 1/4 cup of coconut flakes

- 1/2 cup of Granola

Directions:

1. Combine the acai berries, blueberries, banana, almond milk, honey, and cinnamon in a blender. Blend the mixture until it's creamy and smooth.

2. Place the bowl with the combined mixture in it. Add the granola, coconut flakes, and chia seeds over top.

3. Immediately serve and savor!

SNACK

Edamame

Ingredients:

- 1 cup shelled and boiled edamame

- 1 teaspoon of sesame oil

- 1 teaspoon of soy sauce

- 2 teaspoons Sriracha (or other hot sauce of your choice)

- 1 tablespoon ginger that has just been grated

- Two teaspoons of rice vinegar

Directions:

1. In a medium saucepan over medium heat, warm the sesame oil.

2. Include the edamame to the pan and cook for 3 to 4 minutes, or until the edamame is just starting to brown.

3. Combine the ginger, soy sauce, and Sriracha in the pan.

4. Turn up the heat to medium-high and continue cooking for an additional 5 minutes.

5. Stir in the rice vinegar and simmer for a further 1 to 2 minutes.

6. Right away serve as a side dish or a snack. Enjoy!

LUNCH

Grilled Vegetables and Lentil Salad

Ingredients

- Olive oil, 1 tablespoon

- 1 minced garlic clove

- 1 medium onion, chopped

- 1 Green lentils, 1 cup

- 2 cups of vegetable broth

- Salt & pepper as desired

- 1 yellow bell pepper, thinly sliced

- 1 red bell pepper, thinly sliced.

- 1 cup of halved cherry tomatoes

- 2 teaspoons lemon juice, fresh

-1 tablespoon freshly chopped parsley

- 1 tablespoon freshly chopped oregano

Directions:

1. In a big pot set over medium heat, warm the olive oil. For about 5 minutes, add the onion and garlic and sauté until tender.

2. Add the lentils and bring the vegetable broth to a boil. Once the lentils are tender, turn the heat down to low, cover the pot, and simmer for 20 to 25 minutes.

3. Bring a gas or charcoal grill to a medium heat.

4. After taking the lentils off the fire, season them to taste with salt and pepper.

5. Arrange the lentils, tomatoes, and bell peppers on individual skewers and drizzle with a little olive oil. Grill for 5-8 minutes, or until tender and gently browned.

6. Place the lentils and grilled vegetables in a large bowl. Combine the parsley, oregano, and lemon juice after adding them.

7. Serve warm. Enjoy!

SNACK

Peanut Butter and Apples

Ingredients:

- 2 medium-sized apples

- Creamy peanut butter, 1/4 cup

- Cinnamon, 1/4 teaspoon

- 1 teaspoon of honey

- 1/4 quarter cup of walnuts

Directions:

1. Set your oven to 350 Fahrenheit.

2. Cut the apples into 1-inch cubes after peeling and coring them.

3. Spread cinnamon over the apple chunks in a baking dish.

4. Bake the apples for 25 to 30 minutes, or until they are tender and just starting to turn golden.

5. After the apples have baked through, take them out of the oven to cool.

6. Use a fork to smash the apples in a bowl.

7. Combine the mashed apples with the peanut butter, honey, and walnuts. Mix the ingredients thoroughly by stirring.

8. Spread the mixture evenly in the baking dish.

9. Bake the batter for 15 minutes, or until the top is just beginning to turn golden. Before serving, allow to cool. Enjoy!

DINNER

Rainbow Quinoa with Baked Halibut

Ingredients

- 1 filet of halibut, about 4-6 ounces

- 1 Cooked Rainbow Quinoa, 1 cup

- 1/4 cup of scallions, chopped finely

- Olive oil, 1 tablespoon

- 1 teaspoon lemon juice that has just been squeezed

- 1/2 a teaspoon of dried oregano

- 1/4 teaspoon of sea salt

- Freshly ground black pepper, 1/4 teaspoon

- 1 cup of spinach leaves

- Sliced cherry tomatoes, 1/4 cup

Directions:

1. Set the oven to 350°F.

2. Set the halibut on a baking pan that has been buttered.

3. Combine the cooked quinoa with the scallions, olive oil, lemon juice, oregano, salt, and pepper in a medium bowl.

4. Place the cherry tomatoes and spinach leaves on top of the quinoa mixture that has been spread over the halibut filet.

5. Bake the halibut in the preheated oven for 10 minutes, or until it is thoroughly done.

6. Serve hot. Enjoy!

DAY 7

BREAKFAST

Egg and Avocado Toast

Ingredients:

- A single slice of whole wheat bread

- 1 mature and ripe avocado

- 1 Egg

- Pepper and salt as desired

Directions:

1. The bread should be toasted until golden brown.

2. Using a fork, mash the avocado in a small bowl until it is well-combined. On top of the toasted bread, evenly distribute the mashed avocado.

3. Cook an egg for 5 minutes, or until it is soft boiled, in a small pot of boiling water.

4. Top the mashed avocado with the cooked egg.

5. Add salt and pepper to taste.

6. Enjoy your egg and avocado toast!

SNACK

Greek Yogurt with Berries

Ingredients:

- A single cup of Greek yogurt

- 1/2 cup of berries, either fresh or frozen

- A teaspoon of honey

- 1 teaspoon of chia seeds

- 1 tablespoon of ground flaxseed

- Cinnamon, 1 teaspoon

- 1 teaspoon vanilla bean extract

Directions:

1. Stir the yogurt, honey, chia seeds, flaxseed meal, cinnamon, and vanilla extract together in a medium bowl until thoroughly blended.

2. Gently incorporate the berries.

3. Split the mixture between two bowls, then eat!

4. Enjoy this berry-infused Greek yogurt to help reverse diabetes!

LUNCH

Veggies Roasted and Salmon

Ingredients:

- 2 cups of sweet potatoes cut into cubes

- 1 round zucchini, sliced.

- One red bell pepper, sliced

- 1 slice-able yellow pepper

- 1 onion, sliced into wedges

- 4 minced garlic cloves

- Olive oil, 2 tablespoons

- Salt and pepper

- 6 ounces of skinless salmon fillet

- 2 teaspoons of fresh thyme, rosemary, oregano, or dill

Directions:

1. Set the oven to 400 ºF.

2. On a baking sheet with a rim, arrange cubed sweet potatoes, zucchini, bell pepper slices, and onion wedges.

3. Combine the minced garlic, olive oil, salt, and pepper in a small bowl. Mix thoroughly.

4. After uniformly coating the vegetables, drizzle the olive oil mixture over them.

5. Arrange the vegetables on the baking sheet in an equal layer.

6. Top the vegetables with the salmon fillet.

7. Finish with your preferred fresh herb.

8. Roast in the oven for 20 minutes, or until the veggies are soft and the salmon is fully cooked.

9. Present the fish and roasted veggies hot. Enjoy!

Sliced Apples with Cinnamon

Ingredients:

- 2 peeled and thinly cut apples

- 2 teaspoons of lemon juice that has just been squeezed

- 2 tablespoons of cinnamon powder

- 1 teaspoon of organic, unprocessed honey

Directions:

1. Ensure the oven is set to 375 °F.

2. Let the apple slices sit in the lemon juice that has just been squeezed for 10 minutes. The flavor will become sweeter and more tart as a result.

3. Combine the organic raw honey and cinnamon in a small bowl.

4. After the apple slices have been submerged in the lemon juice, coat them completely with the cinnamon and honey mixture.

5. Spread the apple slices out on a baking sheet that is nonstick. To ensure consistent baking, make sure to space out each one.

6. The apples should be tender but not mushy after 15 minutes of baking.

7. Enjoy the sweet flavor of the warm cooked apple slices.

A drizzle of maple syrup or a dollop of whipped cream can be placed on top of the slices, if preferred, to increase their sweetness.

DINNER

Quinoa burgers and asparagus

Ingredients

- 1/2 cup rinsed uncooked quinoa

- Two sliced garlic cloves

- 1/4 cup onion, minced

- 1 cup of prepared asparagus

- Oat bran, 1/4 cup

- Two teaspoons of almond flour

- 1 teaspoon cumin powder

- 1 paprika teaspoon

- 1/2 teaspoons of sea salt

- Newly ground pepper

- 2 eggs

- Olive oil, two tablespoons

- 1/4 cup crumbled feta

Directions:

1. Bring 1 1/2 cups of water to a boil in a medium saucepan, then add the quinoa. Reduce the heat to low, cover the pot, and simmer for 15 minutes, or until the water is completely absorbed. With a fork, remove from the heat. Place aside.

2. Combine the garlic, onion, asparagus, oat bran, almond flour, cumin, paprika, salt, pepper, eggs, and olive oil in a sizable bowl.

3. Stir in the feta and quinoa, then finish by adding the salt and pepper.

4. Create four burgers out of the mixture.

5. Add the burgers to a sizable nonstick skillet that has been heated over medium heat. Cook for 3 to 4 minutes on each side, or until well heated through and browned.

6. Arrange asparagus and your preferred side dishes alongside the quinoa burgers. Enjoy!

BREAKFAST

Oats for Overnight with Fresh Fruit

Ingredients:

1/2 cup of rolled oats

- 1 cup milk, whether it be dairy, almond, or coconut

-2 tablespoons of honey

- 1/2 teaspoon of cinnamon

- 1 teaspoon of chia seeds

-2 tablespoons Greek yogurt, plain

- 1/4 cup of your preferred fresh fruit (blueberries or strawberries are suggested).

Directions:

1. Combine the oats, milk, honey, and cinnamon in a medium bowl by stirring them together.

2. Wrap the bowl in plastic wrap and place it in the fridge for the night.

3. Stir the fruit, yogurt, and chia seeds in the morning.

4. Share the mixture into the two servings.

5. Enjoy!

Health Benefits:

Because overnight oats are so high in fiber, they can help you manage your diabetes and lower your blood sugar levels. Yogurt's protein content also contributes to energy and satiety. Antioxidants, minerals, and vitamins required for good health are present in the fresh fruit.

Hummus with Crudites

Ingredients:

- 1 can of garbanzo beans or chickpeas

- 2 garlic cloves, peeled and minced

- Tahini, 3 tablespoons

- 3 tablespoons of lemon juice, fresh

- Extra virgin olive oil, 2 tablespoons

- Sea salt, 1/4 teaspoon

- 1/4 teaspoon of cumin powder

- 1 cooked cup of beets or carrots

- 1 cup of precut vegetable sticks, such as carrots, celery, and radishes

Directions:

1. Firstly, rinse and drain the chickpeas. They should be processed in a food processor until they form a paste.

2. Include the cumin, salt, garlic, tahini, lemon juice, and olive oil. Blend everything together completely.

3. Add the carrots or beets to the food processor after peeling and chopping them. Blend the ingredients up to smoothness.

4. Pour the hummus into a bowl, top with the pre-cut veggie sticks, and serve. Enjoy!

LUNCH

Stir-Fried Chicken and Vegetables

Ingredients:

- 1 pound of thinly sliced, skinless, boneless chicken breasts

- 1 red bell pepper, thinly sliced.

- 2 minced garlic cloves

- Vegetable oil, 2 tablespoons

- 1 tablespoon finely minced ginger

- A couple of tablespoons of low-sodium soy sauce

- Rice vinegar, 2 tablespoons

- Honey, two tablespoons

- 1/4 teaspoon of red pepper flakes

- Sliced carrots, 1 cup

- Broccoli florets, 1 cup

- Snow peas, 1 cup

- Sliced water chestnuts, 1/4 cup

- Sliced bamboo shoots, 1/4 cup

- Sliced mushrooms, 1/4 cup

Directions:

1. In a large skillet over medium heat, warm the vegetable oil.

2. Add chicken strips, and allow it cook for about 8 minutes or until golden brown.

3. Include the following ingredients: ginger, soy sauce, rice vinegar, honey, bell pepper strips, carrots, broccoli, snow peas, water chestnuts, bamboo shoots, and red pepper flakes.

4. Stir-fry the vegetables for 10 minutes or until they are soft. Serve hot with brown rice that has been steaming. Enjoy!

Almond Butter and Banana

Ingredients:

- 1 banana

- Almond butter, two tablespoons

Directions:

1. Make thin circles out of the banana.

2. Cover the banana slices with almond butter.

3. Arrange the slices of banana on a platter.

4. Enjoy your nutritious treat!

Benefits: The combination of banana and almond butter, which boosts energy without increasing blood sugar levels and is rich in antioxidants and minerals, can help reverse diabetes. Almond butter also reduces the spike in blood sugar that occurs after meals, which helps to manage diabetes. Additionally, the magnesium in this snack will help to enhance insulin sensitivity.

Broccoli and Sweet Potato with Braised Chicken

Ingredients:

- 1 pound of boneless and skinless chicken breasts (cubed)

- 1 diced medium sweet potato

- 1 head of broccoli that has been cut into florets

- Olive oil, 1 tablespoon

 - Salt & pepper as desired

- 1 teaspoon of ginger root, ground

- 1 teaspoon of garlic-flavored powder

- 1/4 cup of white wine

- 1/2 cup of chicken broth

Directions:

1. Set the oven to 400 ºF.

2. Add salt and pepper to taste and add the chicken cubes to a big bowl.

3. In a sizable oven-safe skillet, heat the olive oil over medium-high heat.

4. Add the chicken cubes and simmer, stirring regularly, for about 3 minutes.

5. Include the broccoli and sweet potato and simmer for an additional three minutes.

6. Include the chicken broth, white wine, ground ginger, and garlic powder and stir to combine.

7. Place the skillet in the preheated oven with the lid on.

8. Bake for 20 minutes while stirring halfway.

9. Warm up the braised chicken with broccoli and sweet potatoes. Enjoy!

DAY 9

BREAKFAST
Avocado, Egg White, and Spinach Omelet

Ingredients:

- 4 egg whites

- Olive oil, 1 tablespoon

- 1/2 cup chopped spinach

- 1/2 cup chopped tomato

- 1/4 Avocado, diced

- 1/8 teaspoon of garlic powder

- A pinch of oregano, dry

- Salt and pepper as desired

Directions:

1. In a medium-sized skillet over medium heat, warm the olive oil.

2. Add the diced tomatoes, diced avocado, and spinach to the skillet. Sauté for two to three minutes, stirring now and then.

3. Whip the egg whites in a small bowl until they are foamy and evenly combined.

4. Place the vegetable-filled skillet with the egg white mixture inside.

5. Season the omelet with salt, pepper, garlic powder, and oregano.

6. Cook the omelet for about four to 5 minutes, or until the bottom is just starting to brown.

7. Gently flip the omelet over, then cook for a further 2-3 minutes, or until the egg whites are set.

8. Serve the omelet warm after cutting it into wedges. Enjoy!

SNACK

Sticks of Celery with Nut Butter

Ingredients:

- 4 celery sticks

- 2 teaspoons of natural nut butter without added sugar

- Honey as desired.

Directions:

1. Wash the celery sticks and pat them dry.

2. Each celery stick should have 2 tablespoons of nut butter spread equally on it.

3. If preferred, lightly brush each celery stick with a teaspoon of honey.

4. Enjoy as a light dinner or a healthy snack!

LUNCH

White Bean and Kale Soup

Ingredients

- Olive oil, 1 tablespoon

- 1 big, diced onion

- 2 minced garlic cloves

- 2 (15-ounce) cans of washed and drained cannellini beans

- Vegetable broth, 4 cups

- 3 cups of finely chopped, rib-free kale

- 1 teaspoon dried oregano

- Salt, 1 teaspoon

- 1/4 teaspoon of black pepper (freshly ground)

- 2 teaspoons of lemon juice that has just been squeezed

Directions:

1. In a big pot, heat the olive oil to a medium-high temperature.

2. Add the diced onion and cook for about 5 minutes, or until tender.

3. Add the garlic and continue to simmer for one more minute.

4. Add the chopped kale, cannellini beans, vegetable broth, oregano, salt, and pepper.

5. After the soup boils, lower the heat to a low setting, and let it simmer for 10 minutes.

6. Turn off the heat and puree the soup in a conventional or immersion blender until it is smooth.

7. Add the lemon juice and taste-test your seasonings before serving.

8. Dish out the soup and savor it!

Greek Yogurt with Berries and Nuts

Ingredients:

- Greek yogurt, 2 cups

-1/4 cup of chopped walnuts

-1/4 cup of chopped almonds

-1/4 cup of chopped pumpkin seeds

-1/4 cup of chopped sunflower seeds

-1/2 cup of fresh or frozen mixed berries

- 1 teaspoon of honey

Directions:

1. Combine the Greek yogurt, honey, chopped walnuts, almonds, pumpkin seeds, and sunflower seeds in a large bowl.

2. Stir everything together until well-combined.

3. Split the yogurt mixture into two bowls, and then top each with a variety of berries. Enjoy!

DINNER

Tilapia Baked with Lentil Salad (For four servings)

Ingredients:

- 4 filets of tilapia

- Olive oil, two tablespoons

- Salt and pepper as desired

- 2 cups of prepared lentils

- 1 thinly sliced medium red onion

- A half-cup of red wine vinegar

- Honey, 2 tablespoons

- 1 tablespoon of Dijon mustard

- 1/2 cup of virgin olive oil

- 2 tablespoons freshly chopped oregano

- 2 teaspoons freshly chopped parsley

- 2 minced garlic cloves

- 1/4 cup feta cheese crumbles

Directions:

1. Ensure the oven's temperature is set to 375 ºF.

2. Arrange the tilapia filets on a parchment-lined baking sheet and drizzle with olive oil. Add salt and pepper to taste.

3. Bake the fish for 15 minutes, or until it is thoroughly done.

119

4. In the meantime, combine the cooked lentils with the red onion, honey, Dijon mustard, extra virgin olive oil, oregano, parsley, and garlic in a large bowl.

5. After the fish has finished cooking, add 2 tablespoons of the lentil salad to each filet. Add some feta cheese.

6. Serve hot. Enjoy!

DAY 10

BREAKFAST

Bowl of Smoothie with Acai Berries

Ingredients:

- 1/2 cup fresh or frozen acai berries

- 1/3 cup of blueberries

- 50 g of strawberries

- 50 g of raspberries

- 1/2 mango

- 1/4 cup almond milk

- A half banana

- 1/2 teaspoon cinnamon powder

- A spoonful of honey

- 1 tablespoon of chia seeds

- 1/4 teaspoon of vanilla extract

- Optional topings include sliced bananas, coconut flakes, and chopped nuts.

Directions:

1. In a blender, combine the mango, acai berries, blueberries, strawberries, raspberries, and almond milk. Blend until combined and smooth.

2. Blend in the banana, cinnamon, honey, chia seeds, and vanilla essence after adding all of the other ingredients.

3. Pour into a bowl, then add any additional toppings.

4. Serve and savor it!

Hummus and Carrot and Celery Sticks

Ingredients:

- 1 cup of matchstick-sized carrot chunks.

- 1 cup of matchstick-sized pieces of celery

- One cup of hummus

- 1 teaspoon of garlic-flavored powder

121

- One teaspoon onion powder

Smoked paprika, 1 teaspoon

Directions:

1. Trim celery and carrots into matchstick-sized pieces after washing.

2. Combine hummus, smoked paprika, garlic powder, onion powder, and other ingredients in a medium bowl.

3. Arrange slices of celery and carrot on a plate.

4. Add plenty of the hummus mixture on top.

5. Enjoy as a side dish or snack.

6. As part of your diet to reverse diabetes, repeat daily.

LUNCH

Avocado and Quinoa Salad

Ingredients:

- cooked quinoa, 1 cup

- 1 chopped avocado

- Sliced cucumber, half a cup

- Chopped half a cup of red bell pepper

- chopped celery in a half cup

- 1/4 cup minced fresh parsley

- 1/4 cup lemon juice, fresh

- Olive oil (extra virgin) two tablespoons

- 1 minced garlic clove

-1/4 teaspoons of sea salt

- 1/4 teaspoon of black pepper, ground

Directions:

1. Combine cooked quinoa, avocado, cucumber, bell pepper, celery, and parsley in a medium bowl.

2. Combine the lemon juice, olive oil, garlic, sea salt, and black pepper in another bowl.

3. Drizzle the dressing over the quinoa mixture and stir to cover everything.

4. Distribute the salad among the four serving plates.

Tips:

Try incorporating 1/4 cup of finely chopped red onion, 1/4 cup of finely chopped toasted almonds, and 1 tablespoon of Dijon mustard into the dressing for an added flavor boost. Enjoy!

Slices of Apple with Almond Butter

Ingredients:

- 2 small apples that have been cored and cut into wedges

- 2 teaspoons of almond butter

- 1 teaspoon of honey

-1/4 teaspoon of cinnamon, ground

- Pure vanilla extract, 1/4 teaspoon

Directions:

1. Set oven to 350 degrees Fahrenheit. On a baking sheet lined with parchment, spread out the apple slices.

2. Blend almond butter, honey, cinnamon, and vanilla in a small bowl.

3. Apply the almond butter mixture on each apple slice with a fork or spoon.

4. Bake for 15-20 minutes in a preheated oven, or until the apples are soft.

Before serving, let the food cool. Enjoy!

Roasted Broccoli and Cauliflower with Turkey Burgers

Ingredients:

- 1 1/2 pounds of ground turkey

- 1/2 diced red onion

- 1/2 cup carrots, grated

- 2 cups cauliflower florets

- 2 cups of broccoli florets

- 2 minced garlic cloves

- 2 teaspoons freshly chopped fresh rosemary

- 2 teaspoons freshly chopped thyme

-2 teaspoons sea salt

-2 teaspoons black pepper

- extra-virgin olive oil, 2 tablespoons

Directions:

1. Set the oven's temperature to 400 F.

2. Mix the minced turkey with the onion, carrot, garlic, rosemary, thyme, salt, and pepper in a bowl. Create four to six patties, then set aside.

3. Arrange the broccoli and cauliflower florets on a sizable baking sheet. Add extra virgin olive oil. Also add salt and pepper as desired. Roast in the oven for 20 to 25 minutes, or until soft and gently browned.

4. Set a sizable skillet over medium-high heat while the vegetables roast. The turkey burgers should be cooked through after being grilled for 5-7 minutes on each side with a tablespoon of extra-virgin olive oil.

5. Serve the roasted broccoli and cauliflower with the turkey burgers. Enjoy!

DAY 11
BREAKFAST

Oatmeal with Berries and Maple Syrup

Ingredients:

- 2 cups of oats cooked in a flash.

- 4 cups of low-fat milk

- 2 sliced, ripe bananas

- 1/2 teaspoon of cinnamon, ground

- 2 teaspoons of maple syrup that is pure.

- 2 cups of your favorite fresh berries (blueberries, raspberries, blackberries, etc.)

Directions:

1. Combine the oats, milk, and cinnamon in a medium pot. Heat over medium – high heat to rolling boil.

2. Stir the oats occasionally as it cooks for 3 to 5 minutes, or until it is well heated through.

3. Distribute the oats among the four dishes.

4. Add sliced bananas, maple syrup, and fresh berries to each bowl.

5. Present and savor!

SNACK

Mixed Nuts

Ingredients:

- Almonds, 1/4 cup

- walnuts, 1/4 cup

- Cashews, 1/4 cup

- Pecans, 1/4 cup

- Macadamia nuts, 1/4 cup

- 1 teaspoon of cinnamon, ground

-1/4 teaspoon of sea salt

Directions:

1. Set your oven to 350 Fahrenheit.

2. In a mixing bowl, add all the nuts and toss to incorporate.

3. Sprinkle with sea salt and ground cinnamon; mix to blend.

4. Arrange the nuts on a baking sheet in an equal layer.

5. Bake for 12 to 15 minutes in a preheated oven, stirring once halfway through.

6. Take the food out of the oven and allow it cool before serving. Enjoy!

LUNCH

Lentil Soup with a Side Salad

Ingredients:

To make the soup:

- Dried green lentils, 1 cup

- 1 diced onion

- 2 minced garlic cloves

- Olive oil, one tablespoon

-3 1/2 cups vegetable stock

- 1 big, diced carrot

-1 chopped celery stalk

- 1 teaspoon each of cumin and oregano

-1/4 teaspoon of red pepper flakes

The side salad will be:

- 1 minced garlic clove

- Olive oil, two tablespoons

- 1 cucumber, sliced

- 4 small tomatoes, cut in half

- 1 tablespoon of white balsamic or white wine vinegar,

- Salt & pepper as desired

Directions:

To make the soup:

1. Heat the olive oil in a pot over medium heat. Add the onion and garlic. For around five minutes, sauté.

2. Include the carrot, celery, cumin, oregano, lentils, vegetable broth, and crushed red pepper. Simmer after bringing to a boil.

3. Let the soup simmer for 25 to 30 minutes, or until the lentils are tender.

4.Puree the soup using an immersion blender to reach the desired consistency.

5. If wanted, top hot dishes with yogurt or fresh herbs.

The side salad:

1. Combine the garlic, tomatoes, cucumbers, olive oil, vinegar, salt, and pepper in a big bowl. Combine by tossing.

2. Serve with soup. Enjoy!

SNACK

Edamame

Ingredients:

-1 cup of edamame in shell

-Olive oil, 1 tablespoon

-50 ml of sea salt

-Black pepper, 1/4 teaspoon

Directions:

1. Turn the oven's temperature up to 350 degrees Fahrenheit.

2. Spread the edamame on a parchment-lined baking sheet.

3. Drizzle olive oil over the dish and season with salt and pepper.

4. Combine by stirring.

5. Bake for 10 to 15 minutes, or until golden.

6. Serve warm, and savor!

DINNER

Salmon baked with Asparagus

Ingredients:

-Fresh salmon fillet, 1 pound

- 1 bunch of trimmed fresh asparagus

- 2 minced garlic cloves

- extra virgin olive oil, two tablespoons

- Salt & pepper as desired

- 2 teaspoons of lemon juice, fresh

Directions:

1. Set the oven to 375°F.

2. Salmon should be placed in a baking dish.

3. Put asparagus next to salmon.

4. Combine the garlic, olive oil, salt, pepper, and lemon juice in a small bowl. Pour over the fish and asparagus after combining everything.

5. Bake for 20 to 25 minutes in a preheated oven, or until salmon is thoroughly cooked and asparagus is tender.

6. Arrange the salmon and asparagus on a plate and top with the remaining sauce.

DAY 12

BREAKFAST
Avocado with Egg Toast

Ingredients:

- 2 slices of whole grain bread

- A half-ripe avocado

-2 teaspoons of freshly chopped cilantro

- Juice made from half lime

- 1/4 teaspoon of sea salt

- Extra-virgin olive oil, 2 tablespoons

- 2 medium-sized hard-boiled eggs

- 2 tablespoons of red onion, chopped

Directions:

1. Heat a griddle or other pan over medium heat.

2. Spread a quarter of the avocado on each slice of bread.

3. Drizzle the slices with the olive oil, salt, and cilantro.

4. Place the bread pieces on the griddle or skillet and toast them lightly for 3 to 4 minutes on each side.

5. Use a fork to mash the hard-boiled eggs after placing them in a basin.

6. Add the mashed eggs and red onion slices to the toast.

7. Pour lime juice over the eggs and toast.

8. Delectably devour the avocado toast with egg.

SNACK

Greek Yogurt and Fresh Fruit

Ingredients:

- 2 cups of Greek yogurt, plain

- 2 cups of fresh fruit, chopped (apples, peaches, berries, etc.)

- Honey, 2 tablespoons

- 1 teaspoon of cinnamon, ground

Directions:

1. Combine the Greek yogurt with the chopped fresh fruit in a medium bowl.

2. Add the ground cinnamon and honey, then whisk to blend.

3. Scoop the mixture into a shallow container, and then freeze it overnight.

4. The next day, serve the fruit and Greek yogurt chilled as a dessert or snack. Enjoy!

Quinoa and Roasted Vegetable Salad

Ingredients:

- Cooked quinoa, 1 cup

- 2 cups of your favorite roasted vegetables (such bell peppers, zucchini, squash, potatoes, cauliflower, onions, etc.)

- 1 medium red onion, diced

- Diced tomatoes, 1 cup

- 2 tablespoons fresh parsley, chopped

- 2 tablespoons lemon juice

- Extra virgin olive oil, two tablespoons

- 1/2 teaspoons sea salt

- 1/4 teaspoons of pepper

Directions:

1. Set the oven's temperature to 350°F.

2. Spread 2 tablespoons of olive oil over the vegetables before placing them on a baking sheet. Vegetables should be lightly browned and soft after roasting for 25 to 30 minutes with sea salt and pepper.

3. Allow the vegetables to cool for 15 minutes after roasting.

4. Combine the quinoa, tomatoes, parsley, diced red onion, and roasted veggies in a big bowl.

5. Add salt and pepper to taste and drizzle with extra virgin olive oil and lemon juice.

6. Gently combine, then serve. Enjoy!

SNACK

Banana and peanut butter

Ingredients:

- 2 ripe bananas.

- 2 tablespoons of peanut butter that is smooth

- 1 spoonful of honey

- Chia seeds, 1 teaspoon

-1/2 teaspoon of cinnamon, ground

- Virgin coconut oil, 1 tablespoon

Directions:

1. Slice the bananas into thin pieces after peeling them.

2. Put the banana slices in a shallow bowl and, using a fork, gently mash them until they form a paste.

3. In a small pan over medium heat, warm the coconut oil.

4. Add the mashed banana to the pan when the oil has melted, and cook it for about 3–4 minutes while stirring occasionally.

5. Add the peanut butter, honey, chia seeds, and ground cinnamon when the mixture begins to boil.

6. Cook the mixture for a further 2 to 3 minutes, stirring now and again, or until it begins to thicken and forms a paste.

7. Remove the mixture from the heat and pour it into a jar.

Take pleasure in this warm banana and peanut butter dish; it is the ideal method to begin reversing diabetes.

DINNER

Stuffed Peppers with Turkey and Brown Rice

Ingredients:

- 6 big bell peppers

- 1/2 pound lean ground turkey

- 1 cup of cooked brown rice

- 1 diced medium onion.

- 2 minced garlic cloves

- 1 ounce can chopped tomatoes

- 1/2 teaspoon of dried oregano

- 1/2 teaspoon of dried thyme

- Olive oil, 2 teaspoons

- Salt and pepper as desired

- Grated parmesan cheese is optional.

Directions:

1. Set the oven to 375ºF. Slice each pepper's top off, then take out the seeds and ribs. They should be put in a baking pan with high sides.

2. In a large skillet over medium-high heat, warm the olive oil. Add the onion and garlic, and cook for 3–4 minutes, or until aromatic.

3. Add the turkey and simmer for about 5 minutes, or until almost done.

4. Add the tomatoes and toss in the oregano, thyme, salt, and pepper. Cook for a further three minutes.

5. Stir in the brown rice that has been cooked. Cook for a further three minutes.

6. Distribute the mixture among the six peppers, tightly putting it within each pepper.

7. Allow it to bake for 25 minutes in a preheated oven. During the final 5 minutes of cooking, sprinkle parmesan cheese on top if preferred. Enjoy!

DAY 13

BREAKFAST
Spinach and Egg Scramble

Ingredients:

- 2 eggs, big

- 1/2 cup of spinach

- 1 tablespoon of coconut or olive oil

-1/4 cup of feta cheese

- 1/4 teaspoon garlic powder

- 1/4 teaspoon onion powder

- Salt and pepper as desired

Directions:

1. Combine eggs, spinach, feta cheese, onion powder, garlic powder, and salt and pepper in a bowl.

2. In a big skillet, heat the oil over medium-high heat.

3. Add the egg mixture to the skillet and cook the eggs for 3 to 4 minutes while stirring regularly.

4. Serve right away. Enjoy!

SNACK

Toast made of Whole Wheat and Nut Butter

Ingredients:

- 2 slices of whole grain bread

- 2 teaspoons of almond or peanut butter

- Cinnamon to taste

Directions:

1. Toast the whole-wheat bread in the toaster until it is just beginning to turn golden.

2. Cover each slice of bread with 2 teaspoons of nut butter.

3. Add a dash of cinnamon to the nut butter.

4. Enjoy your nut butter on whole wheat toast!

Health Benefits:

For people with diabetes, this whole wheat toast with nut butter is a fantastic way to start the day. The whole wheat bread is stuffed with fiber and complex carbohydrates that will keep your blood sugar levels under control. For enduring energy throughout the day, the nut butter adds a beneficial fat to the mixture. Additionally, the cinnamon's addition can lower and stabilize your blood sugar levels. Enjoy!

LUNCH

Avocado-Topped Salad of Kale and Carrots

Ingredients:

- 3 cups of finely chopped kale

- 1 cup peeled and finely diced carrots

- 1 chopped, pitted, and peeled ripe avocado

- Olive oil, 1 tablespoon

- 1 teaspoon lemon juice that has just been squeezed

- 1 tablespoon orange juice that has just been squeezed

- 1 spoonful of honey

- Salt & pepper as desired

Directions:

1. Place the kale and carrots in a large bowl and stir to mix.

2. Combine the olive oil, lemon juice, orange juice, and honey in a separate small bowl.

3. Drizzle the dressing over the kale and carrot mixture and whisk to blend, distributing the dressing evenly.

4. Stir the cubed avocado into the mixture after adding it.

5. To taste, add salt and pepper to the food.

6. Either serve right away or put in the fridge and serve later. Enjoy!

Apple Slices with Cinnamon

Ingredients:

- 4 thinly sliced slices of apples.

- cinnamon, 2 tablespoons

-2 tablespoons of olive oil

- honey, two tablespoons

- 1/4 teaspoon salt

Directions:

1. Set the oven temperature to 350°F.

2. Using parchment paper, cover a baking sheet.

3. Arrange the apple slices on the parchment paper in a single layer.

4. Combine the honey, olive oil, and cinnamon in a small basin.

5. Pour the mixture over the apple pieces.

6. Season the apples with salt.

7. Bake the apples in the preheated oven for 10-15 minutes, or until they are soft and gently browned. Enjoy!

DINNER

Halibut Baked with Rainbow Quinoa

Ingredients:

- Cooked rainbow quinoa, 4 cups

- Olive oil, two tablespoons

- Salt, 1/2 teaspoon

- 1/2 teaspoon of black pepper

- Four 8-ounce fillets of halibut

- 2 minced garlic cloves

- Lemon juice, 2 tablespoons

- Oregano, dry, 1 teaspoon

- 1 tablespoon dried basil

- Black pepper, 1 teaspoon

- 2 teaspoons chopped fresh parsley

Directions:

1. Set the oven's temperature to 400°F.

2. Place the cooked rainbow quinoa on a baking pan and top with a thin layer of olive oil. Add salt and pepper, toss, and bake for 10 to 15 minutes, stirring every few minutes, or until the quinoa is just beginning to turn brown.

3. Arrange halibut fillets on a prepared baking sheet and season with oregano, basil, black pepper, parsley, garlic, and lemon juice. Bake the fish for a further 10 to 12 minutes, or until it is fully cooked and flaky.

4. After the fish has been cooked, flake it and serve it over rainbow quinoa. Enjoy!

DAY 14

BREAKFAST
Greek Yogurt with Berries and Nuts

Ingredients:

- Greek yogurt with no added sugar, 2 cups

- 1/4 cup of chopped walnuts

- 1/4 cup of almonds, chopped

- 1/4 cup of chopped hazelnuts

- 1/4 cup of dried cranberries

- 1/4 cup of blueberries, dry

- 1/4 cup of dried strawberries

- A quarter cup of honey

- 1/4 teaspoon of cinnamon powder

- A pinch of nutmeg

Directions:

1. Combine the yogurt, walnuts, almonds, hazelnuts, cranberries, blueberries, and strawberries in a medium bowl.

2. Add cinnamon and nutmeg and drizzle honey over the dish.

3. Combine by stirring.

4. Spoon the mixture into a serving bowl and take a bite.

5. You can keep any leftovers in the fridge for up to three days by placing them in an airtight container.

Hummus with Carrot and Celery Sticks

Ingredients:

- 4 celery stalks chopped into 4-inch chunks.

- 4 medium carrots, sliced into 4-inch sticks.

- 1/2 cup of hummus from a store

Directions:

1. Turn on the oven to 400°F.

2. Using parchment paper, cover a baking sheet.

3. Combine the celery and carrot sticks with 1/2 tablespoon of olive oil, a teaspoon of salt, and some pepper in a medium bowl.

4. Arrange the vegetables on the baking sheet in a single layer.

5. Bake the vegetables for 20 minutes, or until they are soft and just beginning to color.

6. Take the food out of the oven and let it cool somewhat.

7. Put the hummus on the side and serve the carrot and celery sticks. Enjoy!

Spinach-and-Chickpea Salad Wrap

Ingredients:

- Chickpeas, cooked, 1 cup

- Fresh spinach, two cups

- 1 small onion, chopped

-1/2 cup cucumbers, diced

- Tomato dice, 1/4 cup

- Green bell pepper, chopped, 1/4 cup

- 2 chopped garlic cloves

- Olive oil, 1 tablespoon

- Balsamic vinegar, 1 tablespoon

- 1 teaspoon cumin, ground

- 1 teaspoon of oregano, dry

- Add salt and freshly ground black pepper as desired.

Directions:

Cooked veggies, cooked chickpeas, garlic, olive oil, balsamic vinegar, oregano, cumin, and a pinch of salt and pepper should all be combined in a medium bowl. Stir and set aside.

2. Arrange the spinach leaves on a flat surface, then evenly distribute the chickpea mixture among them.

3. Fold the ends of the leaves together and roll them up like a burrito.

4. Whether at room temperature or chilled, serve. Enjoy!

Apple and Peanut Butter

Ingredients:

- Peanut butter, 2 tablespoons

- Sliced and cored 1 large apple

- 2 teaspoons of cinnamon powder

- Honey, 2 tablespoons

- One teaspoon vanilla bean extract

Directions:

1. Ensure the oven's temperature is set to 350 °F .

2. Combine the peanut butter, honey, and vanilla extract together in a small bowl.

3. Arrange the apple slices in a baking dish and cover with an even layer of peanut butter mixture.

4. Cover the top of the mixture with the ground cinnamon.

5. Allow it to bake for 15 minutes in the preheated oven.

Before serving, let the food cool for at least 10 minutes. Enjoy!

DINNER

Quinoa Burgers and Asparagus

Ingredients:

- Uncooked quinoa, 1 cup

-1/2 cup of asparagus, diced finely

- 1/4 cup of onion, coarsely chopped

- 1 teaspoons of garlic powder

- Oregano, 1 teaspoon

- 1/2 cups of almond meal

- 1 teaspoon sea salt

- 1 spoonful of ground flaxseed

- Olive oil, 1 tablespoon

- 1/4 teaspoon of black pepper

Directions:

1. Set the oven to 350 °F.

2. Combine the quinoa, onion, garlic powder, oregano, almond meal, sea salt, powdered flax seeds, olive oil, and black pepper in a large bowl.

3. Use a fork to mix all the ingredients.

4. Place on a baking sheet in the shape of patties that are approximately 2 inches broad and 1/2 inch thick.

5. After 15 minutes of baking, rotate the pan after 10 minutes.

6. Enjoy it with your preferred condiments!

DAY 15

BREAKFAST

Overnight Oats with Fresh Fruit

Ingredients:

-1/2 cup of rolled oats

-1/2 Cup of skim milk

-1/4 cup of Greek yogurt

-1/4 teaspoon of cinnamon, ground

-1 teaspoon of honey

- Fresh blueberries, 1/2 cup

-1/2 cup of banana slices or other fresh fruit of your choice

Directions:

1. Stir the oats, milk, yogurt, cinnamon, and honey together in a medium bowl.

2. Cover and allow it chill for at least four hours or overnight.

3. In the morning, mix the oatmeal with the fresh blueberries and banana slices. Stir until well-combined.

4. Spoon oatmeal into bowls and enjoy.

Nuts and Dried Fruit

Ingredients:

-1 1/2 cups of raw, mixed nuts (walnuts, cashews, pecans, etc.)

-1/2 cup of unsweetened dried fruit (such as prunes, dates, apricots, cranberries, and raisins).

-1 tablespoon of cinnamon powder

-1 teaspoon of powdered turmeric

-1 teaspoon of ground flaxseed

- Honey, two tablespoons

Directions:

1. Turn the oven's temperature up to 350°F.

2. Add the nuts, dried fruit, cinnamon, turmeric, and flaxseed meal to a bowl and toss to blend.

3. Place the mixture of nuts and dried fruit on a baking sheet.

4. Bake until lightly browned, 10 to 12 minutes, stirring every few minutes.

5. Return the bowl with the nut and dried fruit combination.

6. Drizzle honey over the dish and toss to incorporate it thoroughly.

7. Keep in the fridge for up to two weeks in an airtight container. Enjoy!

LUNCH

Grilled Vegetables and Lentil Salad

Ingredients:

- Olive oil, 2 tablespoons

- White wine vinegar, 1 tablespoon

- 2 minced garlic cloves

- 1 tablespoon Dijon mustard

- 1 cup of cooked lentils

- 1 cauliflower head, divided into florets

- 1 red bell pepper cut into strips.

- 1 slice of sliced zucchini

- 1 red onion, cut into wedges

- 1 tablespoon dried oregano

- 2 teaspoons chopped fresh parsley

- Black pepper, freshly ground, 1/4 teaspoon

- 2 tablespoons of freshly chopped mint

- 2 teaspoons of feta cheese crumbles

Directions:

1. Turn the grill's heat to medium.

2. Combine the olive oil, vinegar, garlic, and mustard in a small bowl. Place the vegetables and lentils on the heated grill after being brushed with the mixture.

3. Grill the veggies and lentils for 8 to 10 minutes, or until they are soft and mildly browned.

4. Combine the grilled veggies, lentils, oregano, parsley, pepper, and mint in a sizable bowl.

5. Completely incorporate the feta cheese.

6. Present warm or cold. Enjoy!

SNACK

Yogurt with Berries in Greek

Ingredients:

- Greek yogurt, 1 cup

- 1/2 cup of berries (strawberries, blueberries, or blackberries), fresh or frozen

-2 teaspoons of honey

- 1 teaspoon cinnamon, ground

- 1/4 tsp. nutmeg

Directions:

1. Combine the Greek yogurt, berries, honey, cinnamon, and nutmeg in a blender or food processor and mix until smooth.

2. The mixture should be divided into two bowls.

3. Immediately serve with additional berries and a dash of cinnamon. Enjoy!

Braised Chicken with Broccoli and Sweet Potatoes

Ingredients:

- 1 pound of skinless, boneless chicken thighs

- 1 large sweet potato, cubed after being peeled

- 1 head broccoli cut into florets

- Olive oil, 1 tablespoon

- Salt, 1/4 teaspoon

- 1/4 teaspoon of black pepper

- 2 minced garlic cloves

- Chicken broth with reduced sodium, 1 cup

- 1 teaspoon of honey

- Balsamic vinegar, 1 tablespoon

Directions:

1. Set the oven to 375°F.

2. In a sizable Dutch oven, heat the oil over medium-high heat. Add the chicken and salt and pepper to taste. Cook for 8 to 10 minutes, or until both sides are golden brown.

3. Fill the Dutch oven with the broccoli florets, garlic, chicken stock, honey, and balsamic vinegar. Stir the mixture.

4. After placing the Dutch oven in the preheated oven, cover it. Cook for 40 minutes while occasionally stirring.

5. Once the sauce has thickened and the veggies are cooked, uncover the Dutch oven and simmer for an additional 10-15 minutes.

6. Arrange the broccoli and sweet potato next the cooked chicken. Enjoy!

DAY 16:

BREAKFAST

Tomatoes, Avocado and Egg White Omelet

Ingredients:

- 1/4 cup of egg whites

- 1/4 cup of tomato dice

- 1/4 cup of avocados, diced

- 1/4 teaspoon of spiced garlic

- 1/4 teaspoon powdered onion

- Salt and pepper as desired

Directions:

1. Turn the heat to medium in a small nonstick pan.

2. In a mixing bowl, beat the egg whites collectively.

3. Add salt, pepper, garlic powder, onion powder, diced tomatoes, and avocado.

4. Move the egg mixture to the skillet.

5. After the bottom side has cooked or turned a light brown, flip the omelet over.

6. Lightly browned the omelet on the other side.

7. Immediately serve the egg white omelet with avocado and tomatoes. Enjoy!

SNACK

Crudites and Hummus

Ingredients:

- 1 can of drained chickpeas

- Fresh lemon juice, 1/4 cup

- 1 minced garlic clove

- Olive oil, 2 tablespoons

- 1 teaspoon of cumin

- Salt and freshly ground pepper as required

-A variety of raw veggies, including carrots, celery, bell peppers, cucumbers, and snap peas.

Directions:

1. In a food processor, combine the drained chickpeas, lemon juice, garlic, olive oil, cumin, and a dash of salt. Blend until smooth.

2. After tasting, adjust the seasonings as necessary. If desired, increase the amount of cumin, salt, and pepper.

3. Place the hummus in a serving bowl and top with some cumin and olive oil as decoration.

4. Serve with a variety of raw veggies, such as carrots, celery, bell peppers, cucumbers, and snap peas. Enjoy!

LUNCH

Vegetables Roasted with Quinoa

Ingredients:

- Undercooked quinoa, 1 cup

- 2 cups of diced mixed veggies, including zucchini, bell peppers, carrots, and sweet potatoes.

- Olive oil, 2 tablespoons

- 2 teaspoons dry herbs, such as basil, oregano, or thyme.

- 1 teaspoon salt, sea

- 1/4 teaspoon black pepper

Directions:

1. Set the oven's temperature to 400°F.

2. On a baking sheet, distribute the diced vegetables and sprinkle with olive oil. Add herbs, salt, and pepper for seasoning.

3. After 25 minutes of roasting, toss the vegetables once.

4. Rinse and drain the quinoa while the veggies are roasting.

5. In a medium saucepan, heat two cups of water to a rolling boil.

6. Stir in the washed quinoa and turn the heat down to low. Quinoa should be cooked for 15 to 20 minutes, or until it is tender.

7. Combine the cooked quinoa and vegetables in a sizable bowl and serve right away. Enjoy!

SNACK

Sticks of Celery with Nut Butter

Ingredients:

-2 stalks of celery

- Natural nut butter, 2 tablespoons

- 1 teaspoon of honey

Directions:

1. Trim the celery stalks into 4-inch sections after washing.

2. Cover the celery with nut butter and drizzle honey on top.

3. Delight in your wonderful and nutritious snack!

DINNER

Tilapia Baked with Lentil Salad

Ingredients:

- 4 fillets of tilapia

- Olive oil, 2 tablespoons

- Salt and pepper as desired

- Green lentils, 1 cup

- 2 cups of chicken broth

- Olive oil, 1 tablespoon

- 2 minced garlic cloves

- 1 teaspoon powdered cumin

- Freshly squeezed lemon juice, 2 tablespoons

- 1/2 cup of chopped parsley

- 1/4 cup of chopped red onion

-2 tablespoons of red bell pepper, diced

- 1/4 cup of goat cheese, crumbled

-2 teaspoons of freshly chopped mint

- Balsamic vinegar, 1/4 cup

Directions:

1. Turn on the oven to 400°F.

2. Spread 2 tablespoons of olive oil over the tilapia fillets before placing them on a baking pan lined with parchment paper. Add salt and pepper to the food. The fish has to bake for 10 minutes in a preheated oven to be fully cooked.

3. Make the lentil salad while the tilapia bakes. Combine the lentils and chicken stock in a medium-sized pot. When the lentils are ready, cook for 15-20 minutes at a simmer after bringing to a boil.

4. Combine the 1 tablespoon of olive oil, the garlic, the cumin powder, the lemon juice, the parsley, the red bell pepper, the red onion, the goat cheese, the mint, and the balsamic vinegar in a big dish. Gently mix in the cooked lentils after adding them.

5. To serve, place the lentil salad on top of the cooked fish.

DAY 17

BREAKFAST

Bowl of Smoothie with Acai Berries

Ingredients

- 1/2 cup of Greek plain yogurt

- Frozen acai berries, 1 cup

- 1/4 cup of almond milk

- 1 teaspoon of honey

Toppings

- 1/4 cup of granola

- Chia seeds, 2 teaspoons

- 2 teaspoons of goji berries, dried

- 2 tablespoons of almonds, sliced

Directions:

1. Blend Greek yogurt, acai berries, almond milk, and honey in a blender.

2. Blend until fluid.

3. Fill a bowl with the smoothie mixture.

4. Sprinkle chopped almonds, granola, chia seeds, and goji berries on top.

5. Present and savor!

Slices of Apple with Almond Butter

Ingredients:

- 2 sliced apples

- 3 tablespoons of almond butter

- 1 teaspoon of honey

- 1 teaspoon cinnamon, ground

- 1/2 teaspoon nutmeg, ground

- A dash of salt

Directions:

1. Set the oven to 350°F.

2. Place the apple slices in a single layer on a baking sheet.

3. Evenly cover the apple slices with the almond butter.

4. Add a drizzle of honey on top.

5. Top with a sprinkle of salt, cinnamon, and nutmeg.

6. Bake the apples in the oven for 10 to 15 minutes, or until tender and caramelized.

7. Let the food cool before serving. Enjoy!

LUNCH

Salmon and Roasted Vegetables

Ingredients

- 1 pound of salmon fillet

- 2 large sweet potatoes, cubed after being peeled

- 2 zucchinis, diced

- 2 seeded and cubed bell peppers

- 2 minced garlic cloves

- Olive oil, 2 tablespoons

- Salt and pepper as desired

- Lemon juice, 2 tablespoons

Directions:

Start by setting the oven to 375°F.

2. Arrange the bell peppers, zucchini, sweet potatoes, and garlic on a baking sheet lined with parchment paper. Sprinkle the vegetables with salt and pepper, drizzle with olive oil, and stir to coat.

3. Top the vegetables with a salmon fillet. Add a lemon juice drizzle.

4. Bake for 25 to 30 minutes in a preheated oven, or until the salmon is cooked through and the vegetables are soft.

5. Serve and eat with lemon wedges!

Peanut Butter with Banana

Ingredients:

- 2 Bananas

- Peanut Butter, 2 teaspoons

- 2 tablespoons of rolled oats

- Cinnamon, 1 teaspoon

- Flaxseed, 2 tablespoons

- Honey, 2 tablespoons

- Coconut oil, 1 teaspoon

Directions:

1. Bananas should be peeled, sliced, and put in a bowl.

2. Melt the peanut butter in a saucepan over medium heat.

3. Add the honey, flaxseed, cinnamon, and rolled oats; whisk to blend everything.

4. After adding the mixture to the bananas, stir them thoroughly to coat them.

5. Add the coconut oil to a nonstick skillet that has been preheated over low-medium heat.

6. Add the banana and peanut butter combination when the coconut oil has melted, and cook for a few minutes or until the bananas are soft.

7. If wanted, top with Greek yogurt, more honey, and a sprinkling of cinnamon while still warm. Enjoy!

DINNER

Turkey Burgers and Fries made of Sweet Potatoes

Ingredients:

- 1 pound of ground turkey

- Freshly ground black pepper and salt

- Olive oil, two tablespoons

- 2 big sweet potatoes, cut and peeled

- 2 teaspoons of thyme leaves, fresh

- 2 teaspoons freshly chopped parsley

- Balsamic vinegar, 2 tablespoons

Directions:

1. Ensure the oven's temperature is set to 375 ºF.

2. Gently combine the ground turkey, 1 teaspoon of salt, and 1/4 teaspoon of black pepper in a large bowl. 4 equal-sized patties should be formed.

3. In a sizable nonstick skillet, heat the olive oil over medium-high heat until it shimmers. Then add the turkey burgers, and cook for about 5 minutes per side, or until golden brown and well cooked.

4. In the meantime, arrange the sweet potato wedges on a sizable baking sheet in a single layer. Add the remaining olive oil to the wedges, season with salt and pepper, then top with the thyme and parsley. Sweet potato wedges should be roasted for 25 minutes, or until crisp and golden.

5. After the turkey burgers are cooked through, add the balsamic vinegar to the skillet and let it thicken for 1 to 2 minutes.

6. Put the balsamic glaze on top of the sweet potato fries and serve the turkey burgers. Enjoy!

DAY 18

BREAKFAST

Bowl of Oatmeal with Fresh Fruit

Ingredients:

- Rolled oats, 1/2 a cup

- 50 ml of skim milk

- 1 cinnamon stick

- 1/4 cup of your preferred fresh fruit, such as strawberries, blueberries, or raspberries, chopped

- Chia seeds, 1 tablespoon

- Honey, 2 teaspoons

Directions:

1. Bring milk to a boil in a small pot.

2. Oats are added, and heat is decreased to a simmer.

3. After about 8 minutes of cooking, mix the oats once or twice.

4. After the oats have finished cooking, take them from the stove and toss in the cinnamon, chia seeds, honey, and fresh fruit.

5. Place in a bowl and savor!

SNACK

Greek Yogurt with Berries and Nuts

Ingredients:

- 2 cups of Greek yogurt devoid of fat

- 12 cup of shelled nuts, such as pistachios, almonds, or walnuts

- strawberries, raspberries, or blueberries, 1/2 cup

- 1 tablespoon of agave nectar or honey

Directions:

1. Greek yogurt should be put in a medium bowl.

2. Add the almonds and berries to the yogurt.

3. Add a drizzle of honey or agave nectar.

4. Combine the yogurt, almonds, and berries by thoroughly mixing everything together.

5. Serve and consume right away.

Wrapped Chickpea Salad with Spinach

Ingredients:

- cooked chickpeas, 2 cups

- 2 cups of spinach

-1/2 cup of tomatoes, chopped

-1/4 cup of red onion, chopped

- Olive oil, 2 tablespoons

- Fresh lemon juice, 1/4 cup

- 1 teaspoons of garlic powder

- Italian seasoning, 1 tablespoon

- Salt & pepper as desired

- 4 whole grain wraps

Directions:

1. Toss the cooked chickpeas with the spinach, tomatoes, onions, olive oil, lemon juice, garlic powder, Italian seasoning, salt, and pepper in a large bowl. Stir everything together thoroughly.

2. As you close the edges, divide the mixture among the four covers.

3. Turn on the medium heat under a skillet.

4. Add two wraps to the skillet and cook for a few minutes, flipping once, until brown. Repeat with the remaining wraps after that.

5. Provide heated wraps and a side of crisp vegetables.

SNACK

Edamame

Ingredients:

- 2 cups of shelled edamame, frozen

- 1/2 cup of fresh garlic, minced

- Lemon juice, 2 teaspoons

- Olive oil, 2 tablespoons

- Salt and pepper, as desired

Directions:

1. Set the oven's temperature to 375 ºF.

2. On a baking sheet, spread the frozen edamame out in a uniform layer.

3. Drizzle lemon juice and olive oil over the edamame after adding the garlic.

4. Stir the edamame to ensure that all of the ingredients are coated evenly.

5. Bake for 20 minutes while stirring once.

6. Add salt and pepper to taste and serve hot. Enjoy!

DINNER

Halibut Baked in the Oven with Rainbow Quinoa

Ingredients:

- 2 halibut filets, each weighing 5 oz./150 g.

- 2 cups raw rainbow quinoa

- Olive oil, 2 tablespoons

- 1 teaspoons of garlic powder

- 1 teaspoon of onion powder

- 1 teaspoon smoked paprika

- 1.2 teaspoons of chili powder

- Salt and pepper as desired

Directions:

1. Set the oven's temperature to 350°F.

2. Using parchment paper, cover a baking sheet.

3. Arrange the halibut filets on the baking sheet that has been ready.

4. Combine the olive oil, smoked paprika, chili powder, garlic powder, onion powder, salt, and pepper in a small bowl.

5. Apply the mixture to the halibut filets, making sure to cover all sides.

6. Bake for ten minutes in the oven.

7. In the interim, make the rainbow quinoa as directed on the package.

8. Combine the rainbow quinoa with the halibut. Enjoy!

DAY 19

BREAKFAST

Avocado with Egg Toast

Ingredients:

- 1 mature avocado

- Whole-grain bread, 2 slices

- 1/2 teaspoon of garlic powder

- 1/4 teaspoons of chili powder

- 1 cup of olive oil

- 1 egg

Directions:

1. Toast the slices of bread until they are crisp and brown.

2. In the meantime, warm the olive oil in a different pan over medium heat.

3. Crack an egg into the skillet and add a little salt and pepper. fry till well done.

4. After peeling, mash the avocado until creamy in a bowl with the chili powder and garlic powder.

5. Place the egg on top of the toast after spreading the mashed avocado on it.

6. Delight in your delicious and nutritious Avocado Toast with Egg for Diabetes Reversal!

SNACK

Almonds and grapes

Ingredients:

- Almonds, 1/2 cup

- 1 cup of grapes without seeds

- Lemon juice, one teaspoon

Directions:

1. Set oven to 350 ºF.

2. Arrange almonds on a baking sheet in an equal layer, and bake for 8 to 10 minutes, stirring regularly, or until they are just beginning to turn golden.

3. Stir the grapes and lemon juice together in a medium bowl to coat them evenly.

4. Chop or crush the cooled almonds into small pieces and stir them into the grape and lemon mixture.

5. Combine by stirring.

6. Serve the grapes and almonds for diabetes reversal at room temperature or refrigerated. Enjoy!

Avocado-Topped Salad of Kale and Carrots

Ingredients:

- 2 cups dried, chopped, and rinsed kale

- 2 cups of grated carrots

-1 avocado, chopped after peeling

- 1/4 cup olive oil

- apple cider vinegar, two tablespoons

- 1 teaspoon of honey

- 1-fourth teaspoon of sea salt

- a sprinkle of black pepper, freshly ground

-1/4 cup chopped walnuts

Directions:

1. Combine the kale and carrots in a big bowl.

2. To make the dressing, combine the olive oil, vinegar, honey, salt, and pepper in a separate small bowl.

3. Add the dressing to the kale and carrots, then toss to coat the veggies well.

4. Gently incorporate the chopped walnuts and avocado.

5. Serve right away or store in the fridge for up to three days. Enjoy!

Cinnamon-Infused Apple Slices

Ingredients:

- 2 apples, peeled, cored, and sliced

-2 teaspoons of cinnamon powder

-2 teaspoons of nutmeg, ground

- 1 teaspoon ginger root

- 1 teaspoon of cloves, ground

Directions:

1. Set the oven's temperature to 350 °F.

2. Arrange the apple slices on a parchment-lined baking pan.

3. Mix the cinnamon, nutmeg, ginger, and cloves in a small bowl until well combined.

4. Evenly distribute the spice mixture over the apple slice.

5. Allow it to bake for 10 minutes in the preheated oven.

6. Bake the slices for a further 5 to 8 minutes, or until the apples are soft and just beginning to color.

7. Serve hot. Enjoy!

DINNER

Quinoa Burgers and Asparagus

Ingredients:

- 1/2 cup raw quinoa

-1 cup chopped, cooked asparagus

-1 egg

- 1 cup of breadcrumbs

-1/2 teaspoon garlic powder

- 1/4 teaspoon of onion powder

- Add salt and pepper as desired

Directions:

1. Set oven to 350 °F.

2. Prepare the quinoa as directed on the package.

3. In a big bowl, combine the quinoa, asparagus, egg, breadcrumbs, garlic powder, onion powder, salt, and pepper.

4. Combine all the components by combining them thoroughly.

5. Create patties out of the mixture and set them on a baking sheet covered with parchment paper.

6. Bake for 25 minutes, or until golden brown, in a preheated oven.

7. Enjoy with lettuce, tomato, and other toppings on a whole grain bun. Enjoy!

DAY 20

BREAKFAST

Avocado, Egg White, and Spinach Omelet

Ingredients

- 3 egg whites

- 1/2 cup thawed spinach, either fresh or frozen.

- 1/4 of an avocado, diced.

- Extra-virgin olive oil, 2 tablespoons

- 1/4 teaspoon of garlic powder

- 1/4 teaspoon of onion powder

- Salt and pepper as desired

Directions:

1. Whip the egg whites together in a small dish.

2. In a nonstick skillet over medium heat, warm the olive oil.

3. Season the skillet with salt and pepper and add the spinach, avocado, garlic powder, and onion powder. The combination should be sautéed for about 2 minutes, or until the avocado is slightly browned and the spinach has wilted.

4. Place the skillet with the egg whites inside. For around 3 to 4 minutes, cook the omelet until the eggs are almost set.

5. After flipping, cook the omelet for one to two more minutes, or until it is firm.

6. To serve, cut the omelet in half. Enjoy!

Toast made of Whole Wheat and Nut Butter

Ingredients:

- Whole wheat toast, 2 slices

- Nut butter, 2 tablespoons

-A pinch of cinnamon powder

- 1 teaspoon of honey

-2 tablespoon of flaxseed meal, ground

Directions:

1. Toast the two slices of whole wheat toast by preheating your oven or toaster to the proper temperature.

2. After the toast has completed toasting, cover both slices with the nut butter.

3. Add some cinnamon to the nut butter's top.

4. Spread out the honey evenly over the cinnamon layer.

5. Cover both toast slices with flax seed meal and push down to make sure it adheres.

6. Arrange both toast slices on a dish and serve.

Enjoy!

LUNCH:

Side Salad and Lentil Soup

Ingredients:

For soup

- Olive oil, 2two tablespoons

- 1/2 cup of onion, diced

- 1 cup of celery, chopped

- 1 cup carrots, chopped

- 1 teaspoon garlic mince

- 1 teaspoon cumin powder

- 1/2 teaspoon coriander powder

- 1/4 teaspoon of turmeric-ground

- Dry green lentils, 2 cups

- Vegetable broth, 6 cups

- 1/4 cup freshly chopped cilantro

For salad:

- ½ cup of cooked quinoa

- 1 cup of diced tomatoes

- 1/4 cup finely minced onion

- 1/4 cup feta cheese crumbles

- Olive oil, 2 tablespoons

-Juice from half a lemon

- Salt and pepper as desired

Directions:

1. In a big pot over medium heat, warm the olive oil.

2. Include the turmeric, cumin, coriander, onion, celery, and carrot. Cook the vegetables for 5 minutes, stirring periodically, or until they are tender and aromatic.

3. Include the lentils and whisk in the vegetable broth. Bring the mixture to a boil by turning up the heat to high.

4. Lower the heat to a gentle simmer, cover, and cook the lentils for 20 minutes, stirring periodically.

5. Stir in the cilantro and turn off the heat. Season with salt and pepper to your taste.

6. In a bowl, mix the quinoa, tomatoes, onion, feta cheese, olive oil, and lemon juice to make the salad. Add salt and pepper as desired and toss to mix.

7. Put the salad on the side and serve the soup. Enjoy!

Carrot and Celery Sticks with Hummus

Ingredients:

- 2 cups of peeled and sliced sticks of carrots

- Celery chopped into sticks, 2 cups

 - Hummus, 1 cup

Directions:

1. Wash the carrots thoroughly after peeling them. Cut into thin, equal-sized sticks.

2. Separate the celery into thin, uniform-sized sticks.

3. Place the carrot sticks and celery in a bowl.

4. Add the preferred quantity of hummus to a bowl.

5. Dip the carrot or celery sticks into the hummus to serve alongside the carrot and celery sticks.

Nutritional Information: This dish is the ideal diabetic-friendly snack because it has a well-balanced amount of fiber, carbohydrates, and protein. Beta carotene and other vitamins and minerals from the carrots and other nutrients from the hummus aid to improve your health and maintain healthy blood sugar levels.

Braised Chicken with Broccoli and Sweet Potatoes

Ingredients

- 4 chicken thighs with no skin or bones

- Olive oil, 2 tablespoons

- Paprika, 1 teaspoon

- 1 teaspoon of garlic powder

- 2Two sweet potatoes, diced

- 1 broccoli head, separated into florets

- 2 cups of chicken broth low in salt

-2 teaspoons of thyme leaves, fresh

- 1 tablespoon balsamic vinegar

- 1 tablespoon of honey

- Salt and pepper as desired.

Directions:

1. Set the oven to 375 ºF.

2. Warm the olive oil in a large skillet over medium-high heat.

3. Add salt and pepper to both sides of the chicken thighs.

4. Add the chicken thighs to the skillet, flipping halfway through cooking for 8 to 10 minutes.

5. Stirring occasionally, simmer the sweet potatoes, broccoli, garlic powder, and paprika for a further 5 minutes.

6. Fill the skillet with the chicken stock, thyme, balsamic vinegar, and honey. Stir everything together.

7. Heat the mixture to a boil, then turn it down to a low simmer and cover. Cook the vegetables for 20 to 25 minutes, or until they are soft.

8. Serve and enjoy.

DAY 21

BREAKFAST

Oats for Overnight with Fresh Fruit

Ingredients:

- 1/2 cup rolled oats, raw

- 1/2 cup of your preferred unsweetened plant milk

- Chia seeds, 1 teaspoon

- Honey, 1 tablespoon

- 1/4 teaspoon of cinnamon powder

- 1/2 cup of your choice of fresh fruit, including blueberries, peaches, apples, and strawberries, diced.

- Optional: shredded coconut, almonds, or walnuts

Directions:

1. Combine the oats, plant-based milk, chia seeds, honey, and cinnamon in a bowl or jar. Stir thoroughly.

2. Include your preferred fruits, chopped, and combine everything.

3. Wrap in cling film and store in the fridge for the night.

4. You can include nuts, almonds, or shredded coconut in the morning before you eat if you like.

5. Take pleasure in your overnight oats cold or heated, as preferred.

SNACK

Mixed Nuts

Ingredients:

- Almonds, 1/2 cup

- Walnuts, 1/4 cup

- Cashews, 1/4 cup

- Hazelnuts, 1/4 cup

- Pecans, 1/4 cup

- 2 tablespoons worth of chia seeds

- 3tablespoons worth of pumpkin seeds

- 3 teaspoons of flaxseed

- Olive oil, 1 teaspoon

- 1 teaspoon of cinnamon, ground

- 1 tablespoon of coconut flakes without sugar

- 1 teaspoon of honey

Directions:

1. Ensure the oven's temperature is set to 350 ºF.

2. Arrange all the nuts on a baking sheet and toast them for 12 to 15 minutes, or until fragrant and lightly browned.

3. Place the bowl of toasted nuts.

4. Include coconut flakes, honey, olive oil, cinnamon, pumpkin seeds, flax seeds, chia seeds, and flax seeds. Mix everything until it is completely coated.

5. Evenly distribute the combined nut mixture onto a baking sheet coated with parchment paper.

6. Bake for 12 to 15 minutes at 350 ºF, stirring regularly, or until aromatic and lightly browned.

7. Allow to fully cool before serving. Enjoy!

Salad with Grilled Vegetables and Lentils

Ingredients:

- Dried lentils, 1/2 cup

- Olive oil, 1/2 teaspoon

- Black pepper, freshly ground, 1/2 teaspoon

- Salt, 1/4 teaspoon

- 1 sliced red bell pepper

- 1 sliced yellow bell pepper

-1 sliced zucchini

-1/2 chopped red onion

- 2 minced garlic cloves

- Lemon juice, two tablespoons

-2 teaspoons finely minced parsley

- Extra-virgin olive oil, 3 teaspoons

Directions:

1. Place the lentils and just enough water to cover them in a small saucepan. Cook for 20 minutes, or

until the lentils are soft, after bringing to a boil and then lowering the heat to a low simmer. Drain, then set apart.

2. Turn the grill's heat up to medium-high.

3. After seasoning the vegetables with salt and black pepper, drizzle some olive oil over them. The vegetables should be grilled for 8 to 10 minutes, occasionally flipping.

4. Toss the cooked lentils, grilled veggies, garlic, lemon juice, parsley, and extra virgin olive oil in a big bowl. Combine by tossing. At room temperature or heated, serve. Enjoy!

SNACK

Greek Yogurt with Berries

Ingredients:

- 2 cups mixed berries (either fresh or frozen)

- Honey, 2 tablespoons

- 1 cup of Greek yogurt

- 1 teaspoon of vanilla extract

- 1 tablespoon of flaxseed, ground

Directions:

1. Place the berries and honey in a medium bowl and stir to blend.

2. Combine the Greek yogurt, vanilla extract, and powdered flaxseed in a another bowl.

3. Distribute the berry-honey mixture among four dessert or parfait glasses in equal portions.

4. Place a quarter of the Greek yogurt mixture on top of each glass.

5. Gently incorporate the Greek yogurt mixture into the berry mixture using a spoon.

6. Prior to serving, chill for two to three hours or overnight. Enjoy!

DINNER

Baked Tilapia with Lentil Salad

Ingredients:

- 2 fillets of tilapia

- Olive oil, 1 teaspoon

- Salt and pepper as desired

-1/3 cup of lentils, raw

- 1 cup of vegetable broth

- Tomato dice, 1/2 cup

- 1 chopped tiny onion

- 1 minced garlic clove

- Olive oil, 1 tablespoon

-1/2 cup of lemon juice

- 2 teaspoons finely minced parsley

- 1/4 teaspoon cumin

- Salt & pepper as desired

Directions:

1. Set the oven to 375 °F.

2. Place the tilapia on a baking sheet, season with salt and pepper, and drizzle with 1 teaspoon of olive oil. Bake the fish for 15 to 20 minutes, or until it is well done.

3. In a medium-sized saucepan set over medium heat, warm the remaining olive oil. For two to three minutes, add the onion and garlic and sauté.

4. Add the vegetable broth and lentils, stir, and then bring to a boil. When the lentils are fully cooked, lower the heat to low and simmer them covered for around 25 minutes.

5. Add the tomatoes, lemon juice, parsley, cumin, salt, and pepper when the meat has finished cooking. Simmer for a further five minutes.

6. Serve

DAY 22

BREAKFAST

Greek Yogurt with Nuts and Berries

Ingredients:

- Greek yogurt, 1 cup

-1/2 cup of assorted nuts, including cashews, almonds, and walnuts

-1/2 cup of mixed berries, such as blackberries, blueberries, and raspberries.

- 1 teaspoon of honey

Directions:

1. Combine the Greek yogurt and honey in a medium bowl.

2. Add the berries to the bowl and whisk in the mixed nuts.

3. Split the mixture between two dishes for serving.

4. Dish out and savor!

SNACK

Apple Slices with Almond Butter

Ingredients:

- 2 two medium apples

- 1/3 cup of smooth almond butter

-1/2 teaspoon of cinnamon, ground

1 tablespoon of optional honey

Directions:

1. Make thin slices of apples.

2. Combine almond butter, honey, and cinnamon in a medium bowl.

3. Evenly smear the apple slices with the almond butter mixture.

4. Arrange the slices on a baking sheet and bake for 10 minutes at 350 °F.

5. Let the slices cool before serving, then savor them!

LUNCH

Quinoa and Roasted Vegetable Salad

Ingredients:

- 2 cups cooked, drained, and rinsed quinoa

- 1 diced onion

- 1 chopped red bell pepper

- 1 diced zucchini

- 1 cup chopped broccoli florets

- 2 minced garlic cloves

- One tablespoon of olive oil

- Balsamic vinegar, 2 tablespoons

- 2 teaspoons freshly chopped parsley

- 1/2 teaspoon oregano, dry

- 1/4 tsp optional red pepper flakes

- 1/4 teaspoon black pepper

- 1/3 cup feta or goat cheese crumbles

Directions:

1. Set the oven temperature to 375 ºF.

2. Arrange the broccoli, zucchini, onion, and red bell pepper on a big baking sheet. Add a drizzle of olive oil and blend by tossing.

3. Roast for 20 to 25 minutes in a preheated oven, tossing halfway through.

4. In the meantime, combine the cooked quinoa with the balsamic vinegar, parsley, oregano, red pepper flakes, and black pepper in a big bowl. To blend, stir.

5. Combine the quinoa with the roasted vegetables by adding them last.

6. Add goat cheese or feta crumbles on top.

7. Present warm or cold. Enjoy!

Nut Butter-Topped Celery Sticks

Ingredients:

- 2 celery stalks, chopped into sticks after being cleaned.

- Almond butter, 2 teaspoons

Directions:

1. After washing, trim the celery stalks into thin, even sticks and set aside

2. Prepare the almond butter.

3. In a bowl, combine the almond butter and stir until it is creamy and smooth.

4. Spread the almond butter over the celery sticks and arrange them on a platter.

5. Either serve right away or keep in the fridge for up to two days. Enjoy your tasty treat!

Roasted Cauliflower and Broccoli with Turkey Burgers

Ingredients:

-2 pounds of turkey meat

- 1/2 teaspoons of garlic powder

- 1/2 teaspoon of onion powder

- 1/2 teaspoons of salt

- Freshly ground black pepper, 1/4 teaspoon

- One-fourth teaspoon paprika

- 1 head of chopped cauliflower

- 1 head of chopped broccoli

- Olive oil, two tablespoons

- Salt & pepper as desired

Directions:

1. Set the oven's temperature to 375 °F.

2. Combine the ground turkey, salt, pepper, paprika, onion powder, garlic powder, and in a big bowl. All materials should be thoroughly combined during mixing. Form into 8 burgers of the same size.

3. Arrange the chopped broccoli and cauliflower on a baking pan. Sprinkle the vegetables with salt, pepper, and olive oil before tossing to coat them well.

4. After the oven has been warmed, put the baking sheet inside and roast for 25 minutes, stirring once.

5. Turn up the heat to medium-high in a big skillet. Burgers should be cooked in a skillet for 8 minutes on each side, or until they reach an internal temperature of 165 degrees F.

6. Arrange the roasted cauliflower and broccoli alongside the burgers on buns. Enjoy!

DAY 23

BREAKFAST

Berry Smoothie Bowl with Acai

Ingredients:

- 2 bananas, frozen

- Acai berries, 12 cup frozen

- 1/2 cup almond milk.

- 2 teaspoon of chia seeds per cup

- 1/2 tsp. ground cinnamon

- Almond butter, 2 teaspoons

- Toppers include some goji berries, sliced bananas, sliced almonds, and shredded coconut.

Directions:

1. Blend the almond milk, chia seeds, cinnamon, frozen acai berries, frozen bananas, frozen almond butter, and almonds until smooth in a blender.

2. Distribute the smoothie between 2 bowls.

3. Add some goji berries, sliced banana, almonds, and shredded coconut on top.

4. Serve right and enjoy.

Edamame

Ingredients

- 1 pound of uncooked edamame beans

-2 tablespoons olive oil

- 1 teaspoon of garlic-flavored powder

- paprika, 1 teaspoon

- Salt and pepper as desired

Directions:

1. Set the oven to 375 ºF.

2. Spread some olive oil over the edamame beans in a baking dish.

3. edamame beans should be baked for 15 minutes, stirring once.

4. Remove from oven and season to taste with salt, pepper, paprika, and garlic powder.

5. Bake the beans for an additional 10 minutes in the oven.

6. Whether hot or cold, serve and savor!

LUNCH

Avocado and Quinoa Salad

Ingredients:

- 1 cup of quinoa

-1/2 cups of corn

-1/4 cup red onion, chopped

-1/4 cup red pepper, chopped

-1/2 diced avocado

-1/4 cup chopped fresh parsley

- 2 minced garlic cloves

- lime juice, 2 tablespoons

- Extra-virgin olive oil, 2 tablespoons

- 1/4 teaspoon cumin

-1/8 teaspoon black pepper, ground

1/2 teaspoons of salt

-1/4 cup of feta cheese in crumbles

Directions:

1. Put the quinoa in a fine mesh screen and rinse it for two minutes under cold running water.

2. Put the quinoa in a small pot. Stir in 2 cups of water. Cover and bring to a boil over medium heat. When the water has boiled, turn the heat down to low and continue cooking the quinoa for 15 to 20 minutes, or until it is fluffy.

3. In the meantime, assemble the avocado, parsley, garlic, lime juice, olive oil, cumin, pepper, and salt in a medium bowl along with the corn, red onion, and red pepper. Until everything is incorporated, stir the ingredients together.

4. After the quinoa has finished cooking, add it to the bowl with the vegetables and seasonings and swirl to blend.

5. Arrange the salad in a serving dish and sprinkle the feta cheese crumbles on top. Serve and savor!

SNACK

Peanut Butter with Banana

Ingredients:

- 2 bananas, ripe

- Peanut Butter, 3 tablespoons

- 1/2 teaspoon of cinnamon

- 2 tablespoons ground flax seeds

- 1 teaspoon of honey

Directions:

1. Use a fork to mash the bananas after peeling them.

2. Add the honey, flax seeds, cinnamon, and peanut butter and whisk to blend.

3. Separate the mixture into two equal halves.

4. Arrange each portion of the mixture on a cutting board or flat plate.

5. Form into two discs that each have a diameter of about 4 inches.

6. Store the discs in the freezer for a half-hour.

7. Savour your chilled Banana and Peanut Butter discs.

DINNER

Baked Salmon and Asparagus

Ingredients:

- 4 fresh salmon fillets (6 ounces).

- Olive oil, 2 tablespoons

-2 tablespoons lemon juice, fresh

- 1/2 teaspoon of sea salt

- 1/4 teaspoon fresh black pepper

- 2 minced garlic cloves

- 1 bundle of trimmed asparagus spears

- 2 tablespoons of freshly grated Parmesan cheese

Directions:

1. Set the oven to 375 ºF. Cooking spray should be used to coat the foil on a baking pan.

2. Arrange the salmon fillets on the lined baking sheet. Sprinkle the salmon with olive oil, lemon juice, salt, pepper, and garlic. Gently work the mixture into the salmon's meat.

3. Position the spears of asparagus around the fish. Add some Parmesan cheese on top.

4. Bake the salmon and asparagus for 15 minutes, or until they are fully cooked.

5. Serve hot. Enjoy!

DAY 24

BREAKFAST

Oatmeal with Berries and Maple Syrup

Ingredients:

- 1 cup rolled old-fashioned oats

- 2 cups of water

-1/4 teaspoon of cinnamon, ground

- 1 teaspoon of pure maple syrup

- 1/2 cup of frozen mixed berries

- Dash of salt

Directions:

1. Combine the oats, water, and cinnamon in a medium pot. Over medium-high heat, bring the mixture to a boil while occasionally stirring.

2. Reduce the heat to low and cook the oats for 5 minutes, stirring periodically, or until they are soft.

3. Switch off the stovetop and stir in the maple syrup.

4. Include a pinch of salt and the frozen berries. The berries should be distributed evenly after stirring.

5. Serve hot. Enjoy!

SNACK

Almonds and Grapes for A Snack

Ingredients:
-1/2 cup almonds, raw

- 1 cup grapes without seeds

- Olive oil, 1 tablespoon

- 1 teaspoon of maple syrup

-1/4 teaspoon of cinnamon, ground

- 1/4 teaspoon of nutmeg, ground

-1/4 teaspoon of sea salt

Directions:

1. Set oven to 350 ºF. Almonds should be uniformly dispersed on a baking sheet. Toast till light golden brown, about 8 to 10 minutes. Let the almonds cool.

2. Clean and dry the grapes. Slit lengthwise in half.

3. Add sliced grapes and roasted almonds to a medium bowl.

4. Combine the olive oil, maple syrup, cinnamon, nutmeg, and sea salt in a separate bowl.

5. After adding the dressing, gently toss the almonds and grapes together.

6. Whether at room temperature or chilled, serve. Enjoy!

This delicious, nutrient-rich salad is a great approach to assist the reversal of diabetes. Grapes add additional fiber and antioxidants, while almonds are a great source of protein, fiber, and healthy fats. This salad is the ideal addition to any diet designed to reverse diabetes!

LUNCH

White Bean and Kale Soup

Ingredients:

- Olive oil, 1 tablespoon

- 1 large, chopped yellow onion

- 2 minced garlic cloves

-3 chopped and peeled carrots

- 2 diced celery stalks

- 2 chopped and peeled potatoes

-6 cups chicken or veggie broth

- 1 15-ounce can of washed and drained cannellini beans

- 1 bunch of kale with the stems cut off and roughly sliced

- 1 teaspoon oregano, dry

- Salt & pepper as desired

Directions:

1. In a big pot, heat the olive oil on medium-high heat.

2. Include the celery, carrots, onion, and garlic. About 8 minutes of sautéing is sufficient to soften and lightly brown the vegetables.

3. Include the beans, kale, potatoes, broth, and oregano. Bring to a boil, then lower the heat to a simmer for about 20 minutes, or until the veggies are soft.

4. Add salt and pepper to taste.

5. If wanted, serve hot over cooked grains or with crusty toast. Enjoy!

SNACK

Peanut Butter and Apples

Ingredients:

- Apples, 2

- Natural unsalted peanut butter, 1/4 cup

- 2 tablespoons of honey

- 2 tablespoons of flaxseed, ground

- Cinnamon, 1 tablespoon

- 1/4 teaspoon of salt

Directions:

1. Slice your apples thinly after washing them.

2. Evenly spread peanut butter over each piece.

3. Top each apple slice with peanut butter-covered teaspoon of honey.

4. Top the honey with the ground flaxseed, cinnamon, and salt.

5. Arrange the slices on a platter and take a bite.

Enjoy this delicious and healthy snack to increase your energy and assist in diabetes reversal.

DINNER

Baked Chicken with Broccoli and Sweet Potatoes

Ingredients:

- 2 chicken breasts, skinless and without bone

- 2 medium sweet potatoes, diced after being peeled

- Olive oil, 2 tablespoons

- 1 teaspoon of garlic powder

-2 teaspoon dried rosemary

- Salt, 1 teaspoon

- 1/2 teaspoon pepper, black

- 1 bunch broccoli cut into florets

Directions:

1. Turn on the oven to 400°F.

2. Put the chicken breast in a baking dish that has been buttered.

3. Combine the diced sweet potatoes with the olive oil, rosemary, salt, and pepper in a basin.

4. Cover the chicken with the sweet potato mixture.

5. Surround the sweet potatoes in the dish with the broccoli florets.

6. Bake for 25 minutes, or until the chicken reaches an internal temperature of 165°F and the sweet potatoes are fully cooked.

7. Add more salt and pepper to taste before serving. Enjoy!

DAY 25

BREAKFAST

Egg and Spinach Scramble

Ingredients:

- 1 tablespoon of olive oil

- 1 cup chopped spinach

- 2 big, beaten eggs

- Salt and pepper as desired

- Optional: 1/4 cup diced cheese

Directions:

1. In a skillet over medium heat, warm the olive oil.

2. Include the spinach and heat for a couple of minutes, or until it softens.

3. Add the eggs and stir the mixture for about 4-5 minutes, or until the eggs are done.

4. To taste, add salt and pepper to the dish.

5. If preferred, include the diced cheese and mix to incorporate.

6. Serve hot. Enjoy!

SNACK

Greek Yogurt and Fresh Fruit as A Snack

Ingredients:

- 1 cup of Greek yogurt, plain

- Freshly squeezed lemon juice, 2 tablespoons

- 1 cup of seasonal fresh fruit, such as blueberries and strawberries.

- 1/4 teaspoon cinnamon, ground

- 1 teaspoon of undiluted honey

Directions:

1. Combine Greek yogurt, lemon juice, and cinnamon in a medium bowl. Blend the ingredients thoroughly.

2. Finely chop the fresh fruit of your choice and stir it into the yogurt mixture.

3. Spoon the yogurt mixture into a container that can close tightly, then place it in the fridge for 30 minutes or until you're ready to serve.

4. Top the yogurt mixture with more chopped fresh fruit, honey, and a dollop of honey.

Enjoy!

LUNCH

Lentil Soup with a Side Salad

Ingredients:

For the lentil soup:

- Olive oil, 2 tablespoons

- A cup of onion, chopped

- 1 cup of celery, chopped

- 2 minced garlic cloves

- 1 teaspoon freshly minced ginger

- 1 teaspoon cumin powder

-1 teaspoon of turmeric-ground

- 1 tablespoon of smoked paprika

- 2 cups of green lentils, dry

- 6 cups of chicken or veggie broth

- Salt and black pepper as desired

For the side salad:

- 2 cups baby spinach

 - 1/2 cup cherry tomatoes

-1/4 cup sliced almonds

- 2 tablespoons olive oil

- 2 teaspoons apple cider vinegar,

- Salt and black pepper as desired

Directions:

To make the soup:

211

1. In a big pot over medium heat, warm the olive oil.

2. Add the onion and celery and simmer for 5 minutes or until tender.

3. Stir in the garlic, ginger, cumin, turmeric, and paprika. Cook for about a minute, or until fragrant.

4. Add the broth and lentils, and then heat to a boil.

5. Lower the heat to a low simmer and cook the lentils for 20 minutes, stirring regularly.

6. Add salt and black pepper to taste, as required.

For the side salad:

1. Combine the spinach, tomatoes, and almonds in a large bowl.

2. Add salt and black pepper to taste and drizzle with olive oil and vinegar.

Serving:

Along with the side salad, serve the lentil soup. Enjoy!

SNACK

Apple Slices with Cinnamon

Ingredients:

- 2 apples, medium-sized

- 3 tablespoons of cinnamon powder

- 1 tablespoon of honey

- 1 teaspoon melted butter

Directions:

1. Set the oven's temperature to 350 °F.

2. Wash and slice apples thinly. Slices should be put in a basin.

3. To make a paste, combine the melted butter, honey, and cinnamon in another bowl.

4. Place each apple slice on a prepared baking sheet after being coated in the cinnamon mixture.

5. To get a golden brown finish, bake the apples for 10-15 minutes.

6. Serve warm, and savor!

DINNER

Stuffed Peppers with Turkey and Brown Rice

Ingredients:

- 4 bell peppers (preferably red)

- 1 cup of brown rice, cooked

- 1 pound of turkey meat

- 1/2 cup white onion, chopped

- 1/4 cup of celery, diced

- 1/2 teaspoon of garlic powder

- Tomato sauce, 1 cup

- Worcestershire sauce, 1 teaspoon

- 1/4 teaspoon of black pepper, ground

Salt as desired

Directions:

1. Set the oven's temperature to 350 °F.

2. Remove the peppers' tops and seed them.

3. In a bowl, combine brown rice that has been cooked with the ground turkey, onion, celery, garlic powder, tomato sauce, Worcestershire sauce, black pepper, and salt.

4. Fill the peppers to the brim with the mixture, then arrange them on a baking tray.

5. Bake in the oven for 45 minutes, or until the turkey is thoroughly cooked and the peppers have softened.

6. Dish out the stuffed peppers and take a bite.

BREAKFAST

Avocado And Tomatoes with Egg White Omelets

Ingredients:

- 2 egg whites

- 1/4 cup avocados, diced

- 1/4 cup tomatoes, diced

- 1/4 teaspoon olive oil

- Salt and pepper as required

Directions:

1. Combine egg whites with a dash of salt and pepper in a small bowl.

2. In a nonstick skillet over medium heat, warm the olive oil.

3. Quickly spread the egg whites evenly in the heated skillet after pouring them in.

4. Cook the eggs for about 3 minutes, or until they are set and slightly browned.

5. Gently flip the omelet over and top one half with chopped avocado and tomato.

6. Gently fold the remaining egg half on top of the tomato and avocado.

7. Cook for another 2 minutes, or until everything is well heated through and gently browned.

8. Place the omelet on a platter and sprinkle more salt and pepper to taste. Enjoy!

Carrot And Celery Sticks with Hummus

Ingredients:

- 2 cups of peeled and sliced carrots

- 2 cups of chopped celery

- ½ cup of hummus

- Salt and pepper as desired

Directions:

1. Set the oven's temperature to 375 ºF.

2. Arrange carrot and celery sticks on a parchment paper-lined baking pan.

3. Bake them for 15 minutes, turning them over halfway.

4. Remove from the oven, then allow to cool.

5. Place the celery and carrot sticks in a serving bowl.

6. Cover the sticks with the hummus.

7. If preferred, season with salt and pepper.

8. Dish out and savor!

Roasted Vegetables and Salmon

Ingredients

- 4 cups of your preferred vegetables, diced into small pieces.

- 2 tablespoons olive oil

- 2 teaspoons of the dried herbs of your choice

- 1 salmon fillet that has been deboned and skinned

- Lemon juice, 1 teaspoon

- Salt and pepper as desired

Directions:

1. Set the oven's temperature to 425 ºF.

2. Fill a big bowl with the vegetables.

3. Drizzle with olive oil and top with your chosen herbs.

4. Continue tossing the vegetables until they have a thin layer of oil on them.

5. Arrange the vegetables in an equal layer on a baking sheet.

6. Top the vegetables with the salmon fillet.

7. Season the salmon with salt and pepper and drizzle lemon juice over it.

8. Bake for 15 to 20 minutes in a preheated oven, or until the veggies are soft and the salmon is fully cooked. Serve hot. Enjoy!

SNACK

Dry Fruit and Nuts

Ingredients:

- 1/2 cup of raw nuts, such as Brazil nuts, cashews, almonds, walnuts, or pistachios

- 1/2 cup of dried fruit, like prunes, dates, apricots, or raisins

- One tablespoon honey

- 1/4 teaspoon of cinnamon, ground

- 1/4 cup of coconut shreds without added sugar

- 1 teaspoon of vanilla extract

Directions:

1. Set the oven's temperature to 375°F.

2. Cover a baking sheet with your preferred nuts and dried fruit.

3. Sprinkle cinnamon over them and drizzle honey over them.

4. Toast for about 10 minutes, or until aromatic and just beginning to brown.

5. Take the baking sheet out of the oven, then let it cool.

6. Add the shredded coconut, vanilla extract, and toasted almonds and dried fruit to a bowl.

7. Combine all the ingredients and mix well to coat everything.

8. Enjoy as a snack or topping for yogurt, cereal, and other nutritious meals.

DINNER

Burgers made of Quinoa And Asparagus

Ingredients:

-1/2 a cup of cooked quinoa

-1/2 cup OF asparagus, diced

-1 egg

- 1/4 cup of whole wheat breadcrumbs

- 1/4 cup of minced garlic

- 1/4 teaspoon of black pepper

- Salt, 1/4 teaspoon

- Olive oil, two tablespoons

Directions:

1. Set the oven's temperature to 350 ºF.

2. Stir the quinoa, asparagus, egg, breadcrumbs, garlic, pepper, and salt together in a medium bowl.

3. Form the quinoa mixture into 8–10 patties with your hands.

4. In a big skillet over medium-high heat, warm the olive oil.

5. Put the patties in the skillet and cook them for 2 to 3 minutes until golden brown on each side.

6. Lay the patties on a baking sheet that has been buttered and bake them in a preheated oven for 10 to 15 minutes, or until fully done.

7. Serve and enjoy with your favorite dipping sauces!

DAY 27

BREAKFAST

Oats for Overnight with Fresh Fruit

Ingredients:

- ¼ cup of rolled oats

- 1 cup of non-dairy milk (or your preferred low-fat milk)

- Chia seeds, 1 teaspoon

- Cinnamon, 1 teaspoon

- 1/4 cup of plain applesauce

- 2 teaspoons of honey (optional)

- 1/2 cup of fresh fruit (such as berries, bananas, and kiwis);

Directions:

1. Combine the oats, chia seeds, and cinnamon in a medium bowl.

2. After adding the milk, stir everything together.

3. Add the honey (if using) and applesauce.

4. Add the fresh fruit mixture.

5. Cover and chill for the night.

6. Take out of the fridge and savor!

SNACK

Crudites and Hummus

Ingredients

- 2 cups drained canned chickpeas

- 3 garlic cloves

- 1/4 cup tahini

- Juice of 1 lemon

- Olive oil, 2 tablespoons

- Salt and pepper as desired

- 2 cups of vegetables, such as broccoli, carrots, celery, and peppers

Directions:

1. In a food processor or blender, combine the chickpeas, garlic, tahini, lemon juice, olive oil, salt, and pepper. Blend until it is smooth.

2. To achieve the required consistency, add one tablespoon of water if the hummus is too thick.

3. Transfer to a bowl and top with crudites. Enjoy!

LUNCH
Wrapped Chickpea Salad with Spinach

Ingredients:

- 2 cups of cooked chickpeas

- 2 cups of new spinach leaves

- Olive oil, 2 tablespoons

- 2 minced garlic cloves

- 1/2 teaspoon cumin, ground

- 1/4 teaspoon of sea salt

- 1/4 teaspoon of black pepper, ground

- Juice from a half-lemon.

- 2 tortillas made of whole wheat

Directions:

1. Toss the cooked chickpeas, fresh spinach leaves, olive oil, garlic, cumin, salt, and pepper in a medium bowl.

2. Combine the lemon juice and two tablespoons of the olive oil in a small bowl.

3. Warm the tortillas in a dry skillet over medium-high heat. Till they are just faintly browned, flip the tortillas every few seconds.

4. Cover one side of the tortillas equally with the chickpea mixture before drizzling the lemon juice and olive oil mixture over the top.

5. Divide the tortilla in half, then serve right away. Enjoy!

SNACK

Yogurt with Berries in Greek

Ingredients:

- 1 cup of unflavored Greek yogurt

- 1/2 cup of raspberries, either fresh or frozen

- 1/2 cup of blueberries, either fresh or frozen

- A tablespoon of honey

- 1 teaspoon of cinnamon powder

Directions:

1. Add the honey and cinnamon to the Greek yogurt in a bowl.

2. Include the blueberries and raspberries in the mixture.

3. Fill each bowl with the Greek yogurt and berry combination. Enjoy!

Benefits:

Probiotic bacteria included in Greek yogurt have been shown to lower inflammation and aid in type 2 diabetes reversal. The berries and honey are organic sources of antioxidants that lower inflammation and aid in the treatment of type 2 diabetes. The anti-inflammatory and anti-diabetic effects of cinnamon are provided. With the help of this recipe, you can help reverse type 2 diabetes while enjoying a tasty, healthful snack.

DINNER

Halibut Baked with Rainbow Quinoa

Ingredients:

- Extra-virgin olive oil, 2 tablespoons

- 2 minced garlic cloves

- 1 teaspoon of paprika

- 1/2 teaspoons of salt

- 1/4 teaspoon of freshly ground pepper

-2 fillets of halibut

- 1/4 cup of white wine

- Cooked rainbow quinoa, 2 cups

-2 tablespoons fresh parsley, minced

Directions:

1. Set the oven to 375°F.

2. Combine the olive oil, garlic, paprika, salt, and pepper in a small bowl. Rub the halibut fillets with the mixture all over.

3. Set the fillets on a baking sheet covered with parchment paper. White wine should be added to the pan with the fish. Depending on the thickness of the fish, bake for 15-20 minutes or until flaky.

4. Prepare the quinoa per the directions on the package while the fish bakes.

5. After the fish has baked, place it on a serving tray and garnish with cooked rainbow quinoa and finely chopped parsley. Serve alongside a side dish of your preferred vegetables. Enjoy!

BREAKFAST

Avocado Toast with Egg

Ingredients:

- 1 pitted and mashed ripe avocado

- 2 eggs, big

- 2 slices of whole wheat bread

- Olive oil, 1 teaspoon

- Salt and pepper as desired

- 1/4 teaspoons of ground coriander and smoked paprika, respectively

- Fresh cilantro sprigs (optional)

Directions:

1. In a skillet over medium heat, warm the olive oil.

2. Crack an egg into each skillet, season with salt and pepper, and cook for two to three minutes or until set.

3. In the meantime, combine the mashed avocado, coriander, and smoked paprika in a medium bowl.

4. Top the toast slices with the mashed avocado.

5. Top each piece of toast with a cooked egg.

6. Garnish with cilantro sprigs if you so wish. Serve and Enjoy!

SNACK

Celery Sticks with Nut Butter

Ingredients:

- 4 stalks of celery

- 3 tablespoons of the nut butter of your choice

-A dash of cinnamon, if desired

-A small amount of salt

Directions:

1. Wash and pat celery dry. Make four cuts after that.

2. Spread the celery out on a platter.

3. Each celery stick should have 1 teaspoon of nut butter on it.

4. As an optional garnish, you might add a little sea salt and cinnamon.

5. Serve and savor!

LUNCH

Vegetables Roasted with Quinoa

Ingredients:

- 1 cup of quinoa

- Olive oil, 1 tablespoon

- 1 diced onion

- 2 minced garlic cloves

-1/2 chopped red pepper

-1/2 sliced zucchini

-1/2 chopped eggplant

- 1 cup of cherry tomatoes

- 1 teaspoon cumin, ground

- 1/2 teaspoon of paprika

- 1/4 teaspoon of black pepper

- 2 teaspoons chopped fresh parsley

-1/4 cup of feta cheese in crumbles

- Juice made from half a lemon

Directions:

1. Set the oven's temperature to 400 ºF.

2. When the quinoa is prepared, follow the directions on the package and set it aside.

3. Spread a generous layer of olive oil over the entire assortment of vegetables. Add some pepper, paprika, and cumin.

4. To roast veggies, place them in the oven for 25 to 30 minutes, stirring halfway through, or until they are soft.

5. Combine the quinoa, roasted veggies, parsley, feta cheese, and lemon juice in a big bowl. Completely combine.

6. Serve hot and savor!

SNACK

Apple and Peanut Butter

Ingredients:

- 2 diced and cored apples

- 2 tablespoons of smooth peanut butter, if possible.

- Honey, 2 tablespoons

- 2 tablespoons heavy whipping cream

- Nutmeg, 1 teaspoon

- 1/2 teaspoon of cinnamon powder

- 1/4 teaspoon of cardamom powder

Directions:

1. Combine the heavy cream, honey, peanut butter, and diced apples in a medium basin. Mix everything together with a spoon until it is thoroughly combined.

2. Add the nutmeg, cinnamon, and cardamom, stirring to incorporate all the ingredients.

3. Divide the dish into four portions and serve it warm. Enjoy!

DINNER

Braised Chicken with Broccoli and Sweet Potatoes

Ingredients:

- Olive oil, two tablespoons

- 1/2 medium sweet onion, diced

- 2 minced garlic cloves

- Cut up four chicken breasts into 1-inch cubes.

- 1/2 teaspoon of smoked paprika

-1/2 teaspoon of dried oregano

- 1/4 teaspoon coriander powder

- A pinch of salt

- 1/4 teaspoon of black pepper (freshly ground)

- 2 cups of chicken broth low in salt

- 2 medium sweet potatoes, diced after being peeled
- 2 cups of broccoli florets

Directions:

1. Set the oven's temperature to 375 ºF.

2. The olive oil should be warmed in a large skillet over medium heat. Cook the onion and garlic for about 4 minutes, or until they are tender and fragrant.

3. Add the chicken cubes and season with salt, pepper, paprika, oregano, and coriander. Cook for about 5 minutes, tossing periodically, or until chicken is thoroughly cooked.

4. Place the chicken, onions, and chicken broth in a 9x13" baking dish. Stir in the sweet potatoes after adding them.

5. Bake the dish for 25 minutes in a preheated oven while it is covered with foil.

6. Take off the foil, toss in the broccoli florets, and bake for a further 10 minutes, or until the chicken is thoroughly cooked and the broccoli is soft.

7. Serve hot and savor!

BREAKFAST

Smoothie Bowl with Acai Berries

Ingredients:

- 1 packet of acai berries, frozen

- 1 banana, ripe

- Almond milk, 1/2 cup

- Honey, 1 tablespoon

-1/2 cup of blueberries, frozen

-1/4 cup of almonds, chopped

- 1teaspoon of chia seeds

- Greek yogurt, 1/4 cup

- 1/4 cup of granola

- Cinnamon, 1/2 teaspoon

Directions:

1. In a blender, combine the acai berries, banana, almond milk, and honey; process until smooth.

2. Put the ingredients in a bowl.

3 Add cinnamon, Greek yogurt, oats, chopped almonds, and blueberries.

4. Continue blending to obtain the required consistency.

5. Dish it up and enjoy!

Apple Slices with Almond Butter

Ingredients

- 2 big apples

- 4 tablespoons of unsalted almond butter

- 2 tablespoons of cinnamon, ground

-2 teaspoons of honey

Directions:

1. Set the oven to 375 ºF.

2. Cut apples into thin (about 1/4 inch thick) slices.

3. Arrange the apple slices on a parchment-lined baking pan.

4. Combine the almond butter, honey, cinnamon, and in a small bowl.

5. Cover the apple slices with the almond butter mixture. Make sure to evenly cover them.

6. Allow it to bake until golden brown, about 10 to 15 minutes.

7. Enjoy while serving warm or at room temperature!

Avocado-Topped Salad of Kale and Carrots

Ingredients

- 3 cups of finely chopped kale

- 2 carrots, grated

- 1 diced avocado

-2 tablespoons olive oil

- 1 tablespoon lemon juice, fresh

- 1 tablespoon of dijon mustard

- Salt and pepper as desired

Directions:

1. Combine the greens and carrots in a bowl.

2. Combine the olive oil, lemon juice, dijon mustard, salt, and pepper in another bowl.

3. Drizzle the salad dressing over the kale and carrots, then toss to blend.

4. Stir gently until mixed after adding the chopped avocado.

5. Serve cold and savor!

Banana And Peanut Butter

Ingredients:

- 1 banana, ripe

- Natural Peanut Butter, 2 teaspoons

Directions:

1. Slice the banana into tiny pieces after peeling it.

2. Evenly smear the pieces with peanut butter.

3. Arrange the slices on a baking sheet and bake for about 10 minutes in a 350°F preheated oven.

4. Take the bananas out of the oven, let them cool, and then enjoy.

DINNER

Tilapia Baked with Lentil Salad

Ingredients:

- 2 fillets of tilapia

- 2 tablespoons lemon juice, fresh

- 2 minced garlic cloves

- Extra-virgin olive oil, 2 tablespoons

-2 teaspoon freshly chopped parsley

- 1 teaspoon of dried oregano

- A dash of salt

- Any type of lentil salad you choose.

Directions:

1. Set the oven to 375°F.

2. Use extra virgin olive oil to grease a baking dish.

3. Fillets of tilapia are added to the meal.

4. Season the fish with sea salt, parsley, oregano, extra virgin olive oil, lemon juice, and garlic.

5. Bake for 15-20 minutes in a preheated oven, or until the fish flakes easily with a fork.

6. Make your preferred lentil salad and put it on the table with the fish. Enjoy!

DAY 30

BREAKFAST
Bowl of Oatmeal with Fresh Fruit

Ingredients:

- 1 cup of rolled oats

- Water, 1¼ cup

- Honey, 1 spoonful

-1/4 teaspoon of cinnamon, ground

- Coconut oil, 1 teaspoon

- Blueberries, 1/2 cup

-1/2 cup of diced fresh fruit (apples, strawberries, bananas, etc.)

Directions:

1. Heat the oats and water in a small saucepan over medium-high heat. Stirring regularly, bring the mixture to a gentle boil.

2. Lower the heat to a low simmer, stirring regularly, for 5 minutes, or until the oats are thick and mushy.

3. Turn off the heat and stir in the coconut oil, honey, and cinnamon. Mix everything together by stirring.

4. Transfer the oats into a bowl and garnish with blueberries, fresh fruit dice, or any other extras you choose. Serve hot. Enjoy!

SNACK

Mixed Nuts

Ingredients:

- 2 cups of nuts

- Pecans, 2 cups

- 2 cups of almonds

- Hazelnuts, 2 cups

- 1 tablespoon of honey

- Extra-virgin olive oil, 2 tablespoons

- 1 teaspoon of ginger powder

- 1 teaspoon cinnamon powder

- 1/4 teaspoon of cayenne pepper

- A pinch of salt

- ¼ teaspoon of freshly ground black pepper

Directions:

1. Line a baking sheet with parchment paper and preheat the oven to 350°F.

2. Combine walnuts, pecans, almonds, and hazelnuts with honey, olive oil, ginger, cinnamon, cayenne, salt, and pepper in a larger bowl.

3. Cover the baking sheet with the nut mixture.

4. Bake the nuts for 8 to 10 minutes, stirring halfway through, or until they are fragrant and golden brown.

5. Allow to cool and keep for up to a week in an airtight container. Enjoy!

Grilled Vegetables and Lentil Salad

Ingredients:

- 2 cups of cooked lentils

- 1 large eggplant, cut into circle about 1/2 inch thick.

- 1 large zucchini, cut into circle about 1/2 inch thick.

- 1 sliced, seeded, and cored red bell pepper

- Olive oil, 2 tablespoons

- 1 teaspoon of garlic powder

- 1 tablespoon cumin

- 1 teaspoon of turmeric

- Salt and pepper as desired

Dressing:

-2 teaspoon extra virgin olive oil

- 1 teaspoon lemon juice that has just been squeezed

- 1 tablespoon freshly chopped parsley

- 1 teaspoon of garlic, minced

- Salt and pepper as desired

Directions:

1. Turn on the medium-high heat and prepare a grill or grill pan.

2. Season the bell pepper, eggplant, and zucchini pieces with salt, pepper, turmeric, garlic powder, and olive oil.

3. Grill the vegetables for about 5 minutes per side, tossing once, until they are softened and just beginning to brown.

4. Combine the cooked lentils with the grilled veggies on a platter.

5. Combine the olive oil, lemon juice, parsley, garlic, salt, and pepper in a small bowl.

6. Drizzle the salad with the dressing and enjoy!

SNACK

Hummus and Celery Sticks

Ingredients:

- Two big carrots

- 2 substantial celery stalks

- 2 tablespoons of hummus that has been made.

Directions:

1. Cut the celery and carrots into thin sticks after washing and peeling them.

2. The carrot and celery sticks should be put in a bowl.

3. Use a spoon or a whisk to combine the two tablespoons of prepared hummus in a different bowl so that it becomes a smooth dip.

4. Arrange the carrot and celery sticks on a platter and serve them with the hummus dip. Enjoy!

DINNER

Turkey Burgers and Fries Made Of Sweet Potatoes

Ingredients:

- 1 pound turkey ground

- 2 onions, chopped finely

- 1/4 cup of fresh parsley, chopped finely

- A pinch of garlic powder

- 1/2 paprika teaspoon

- 1/4 teaspoon freshly ground pepper

- 2 sweet potatoes, thinly sliced.

- Olive oil, two tablespoons

- A pinch of salt

Directions:

1. Set the oven to 425 °F.

2. Combine the ground turkey, scallions, parsley, garlic powder, paprika, and pepper in a big basin. 4 equal-sized patties should be formed.

3. Turn up the heat to medium-high in a sizable skillet. The turkey patties should be cooked through after about 8 minutes on each side.

4. Make the sweet potato fries while the burgers are cooking. On a baking pan, arrange the sweet potato slices. Salt and olive oil are drizzled on top.

5. Bake for about 20 minutes, flipping once, or until the fries are crispy in the preheated oven.

6. Put the sweet potato fries alongside the turkey burgers. Enjoy!